WESTERN NEVADA COLLEGE

3 1439 00079 6642

D0214187

DATE DUE

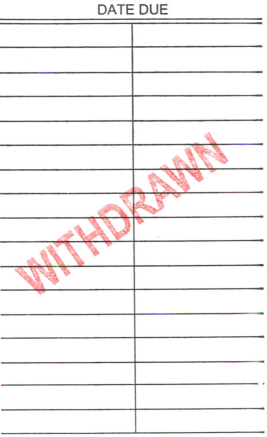

DEMCO, INC. 38-2931

LIBRARY & MEDIA SERVICES
WESTERN NEVADA COLLEGE
2201 WEST COLLEGE PARKWAY
CARSON CITY, NV 89703

American Nursing

American Nursing

A History of Knowledge, Authority,
and the Meaning of Work

WNC
RT
4
D357
2010
MAR 31 '11

PATRICIA D'ANTONIO

The Johns Hopkins University Press

Baltimore

© 2010 The Johns Hopkins University Press
All rights reserved. Published 2010
Printed in the United States of America on acid-free paper
9 8 7 6 5 4 3 2 1

The Johns Hopkins University Press
2715 North Charles Street
Baltimore, Maryland 21218-4363
www.press.jhu.edu

Library of Congress Cataloging-in-Publication Data

D'Antonio, Patricia, 1955–
  American nursing : a history of knowledge, authority, and the meaning of work /
Patricia D'Antonio.
      p. ; cm.
  Includes bibliographical references and index.
  ISBN-13: 978-0-8018-9564-7 (hardcover : alk. paper)
  ISBN-10: 0-8018-9564-2 (hardcover : alk. paper)
  ISBN-13: 978-0-8018-9565-4 (pbk. : alk. paper)
  ISBN-10: 0-8018-9565-0 (pbk. : alk. paper)
  1. Nursing—United States—History. I. Title.
  [DNLM: 1. History of Nursing—United States. 2. History, 19th Century—
United States. 3. History, 20th Century—United States. 4. Nurse's Role—history—
United States. WY 11 AA1 D194a 2010]
  RT4.D357 2010
  610.730973—dc22   2009037380

A catalog record for this book is available from the British Library.

Special discounts are available for bulk purchases of this book. For more information,
please contact Special Sales at 410-516-6936 or specialsales@press.jhu.edu.

The Johns Hopkins University Press uses environmentally friendly book materials,
including recycled text paper that is composed of at least 30 percent post-consumer
waste, whenever possible. All of our book papers are acid-free, and our jackets and
covers are printed on paper with recycled content.

CONTENTS

ACKNOWLEDGMENTS

T HIS STUDY HAS ITS ROOTS in a simple request made years ago that I construct an essay reviewing research in the history of nursing. That the project has grown into something much larger is a testament to the advice and support of an extraordinary group of individuals whose have helped in immeasurable ways. I have accrued many debts, and the first are literal. My intent to tell a story about the history of nursing across the United States was an expensive one, and I am particularly grateful for a research grant from the Xi Chapter of Sigma Theta Tau, the Nursing Society Research Award from the American Association for the History of Nursing, and the Barbara Brodie Nursing History Fellowship from the University of Virginia. These awards made my initial travels possible. They also laid the groundwork for a grant from the National Library of Medicine (#1 G13 LM08199-01) that generously covered more travel and, just as important, time to begin drafting this book. A Penn Humanities Forum Mellon Faculty Research Fellowship supported the construction of the first chapter on the origins of trained nursing, and I am grateful for the critiques and suggestions of the colleagues I met there both from within and outside the University of Pennsylvania. Finally, a fellowship from the National Endowment for the Humanities (FA-53834-08) allowed me the incredible luxury of a sustained period of time when my only responsibility was to finish this book; I thank Lois Evans for making it possible for me to have this time.

Over the years I have worked on this study, I have found myself surrounded by friends and colleagues generously offering advice, suggestions, and resources. I am grateful to Carla Schissel, whose own work on Georgia's nurses has been invaluable to me, for sharing some of her data, her knowledge of sources, her critiques, and her gracious hospitality. I am also grateful to Anita Martin at Atlanta's Auburn Avenue Research Library on African American Culture and History, who allowed me access to the unprocessed papers of the National Grady Nurses Conclave, and to Joyce Ojala, who took time out of her busy schedule to take me on a tour of Grady Memorial Hospital.

In North Carolina, Janna Dieckmann steered me toward data on the two separate and segregated nurses' associations; this book would be poorer but for her advice that their stories needed telling. As I moved west, Elaine Sorensen Marshall, Jill Mulvay Derr, Carol Madsen, and Jennifer Reeder helped me understand the religious and social background of the Church of Jesus Christ of Latter-day Saints. I also thank Marilyn Flood for generously sharing her knowledge of California's nursing history; Valerie Wheat, the archivist at the University of California, San Francisco's library; and David Kessler at the Bancroft Library at the University of California, Berkeley, for unearthing letters and diaries that have enriched my own work.

I am especially grateful to those who took time from their own research to critique mine. Naomi Rogers helped me reshape an early draft of my story about nurses as wives and mothers, and advice from Karen Flynn sharpened my thinking about the intersections of gender and race in nursing. Matthew Creighton and Hiram Beltran-Sanchez, then graduate students in the Population Studies Center at the University of Pennsylvania, came to my rescue when I realized that extracting useable samples from the IPUMS database was not as simple as I thought; and Jean Whelan helped me think through the analyses of the early twentieth-century data. Susan Reverby supported this project from the beginning, and my book is richer for her critiques and suggestions.

The Barbara Bates Center for the Study of the History of Nursing at the University of Pennsylvania has been my intellectual home for over two decades, and I remain grateful for the support, collegiality, good counsel, and friendships I have found there. Cynthia Connolly and Karen Buhler-Wilkerson both read versions of the entire manuscript, and their comments and suggestions sharpened my sense of context, strengthened my arguments and, although I own any remaining errors, saved me from some dreadful mistakes. Julie Fairman, Ellen Baer, and Barbra Mann Wall have patiently listened to me—in formal and informal sessions—endlessly discussing various aspects of this study from its earliest inception through to the final product. My greatest debt is to Joan Lynaugh, not only for constantly reading different versions of this manuscript but also for the exacting standards and innumerable kindnesses that have always shown me what it means to be a true scholar, nurse, and friend.

As this study draws to a close, I thank Jacqueline Wehmueller at the Johns Hopkins University Press, who always made me feel as if I was her only author. As always, my husband, Joseph D'Antonio, deserves much more than my expressions of sincere gratitude for his constant encouragement, perspective, patience, and unfailing optimism. His and my son Frank's pride in my work has always sustained me.

Portions of the following articles are used with the permissions of the publishers: "Counting Nurses: The Power of Historical Census Data," *Journal of Clinical Nursing* 18 (2009): 2717–24; "Nurses—and Wives and Mothers: Women and the Latter-Day Saints Training School's Class of 1919," *Journal of Women's History* 19, no. 3 (2007): 112–36; "Women, Nursing, and Baccalaureate Education in Twentieth Century America," *Journal of Nursing Scholarship* 36, no. 4 (2004): 379–84; and "'All a Woman's Life Can Bring': The Domestic Roots of Nursing in Philadelphia, 1830–1885," *Nursing Research* 36, no. 1 (1987): 12–17.

F ULL DISCLOSURE: I am a nurse as well as an historian. I had never dreamed of becoming a nurse as a child. On the contrary, I entered college with vague ideas about constructing a literary life as an English or history major. I was not without talent in these areas, but I quickly realized that this path to the economic independence I wanted—and needed—would be very long and arduous. I surveyed my options. I did not feel I had the patience to teach or what I believed to be the harder edge necessary to succeed in business. That, in my particular college, left nursing. I transferred as a sophomore for very pragmatic reasons. I fell in love with psychiatric nursing as a senior. I have never looked back.

This book is certainly framed by this experience, but I trust that my later training as a historian prevents its being limited by it. My eventual return to history in graduate school allowed me to recognize how, over time, different nurses told different stories. Some told ones about childhood dreams, and others spoke about frustrated ambitions. My training also gave me the analytic tools to think more broadly about the meanings of all these stories. On one level, then, *American Nursing* is about the history of nurses as told through their stories. It is a history of difference and diversity. As such, it captures the myriad ways in which women and some men reframed the most traditional of gendered expectations— that of caring for the sick—in ways that allowed them to renegotiate the terms of some of their experiences and to reshape their own sense of worth, value, and power.

But on another level, this book is also a history of women. It considers the experiences of nurses—women from different backgrounds, with different ambitions and different life experiences—to capture the possibilities, power, and problems inherent in the ways women (and some men) considered their choices, defined their work, and lived their lives. It builds on data sources such as diaries, nursing alumni association surveys, and oral histories that tell stories of lives lived over time rather than just at particular moments in time. It also attends to the inter-mingled experiences of women's home work, care work, community work, and paid work. Like Laurel Thatcher Ulrich's study of Martha Ballard, the midwife in *A Midwife's Tale* (New York: Knopf, 1990) and Emily Abel's work on the experiences of women caring for sick kin in *Hearts of Wisdom: American Women Caring for Kin, 1850–1940* (Cambridge: Harvard University Press, 2000), my book emphasizes the si-multaneity of lives lived as mothers, midwives, nurses, spouses, neigh-bors, and friends.

My book also draws on historical scholarship that rethinks work as all paid and unpaid endeavors that help both an individual and a family maintain social and economic stability. These perspectives have dra-matically enriched historians' sense of the worth of different forms of dif-ferent women's work in different kinds of locations. Women's housework, their work rearing children and caring for sick family members, and their unpaid work on their family's farms and businesses are increas-ingly conceptualized as equal to and as meaningful as paid work in professional offices, on the factory floor, or about the hospital ward.[1] But the experiences of white men, white women professionals, or white working-class women are no longer normative. Broader questions probe how race, religion, place, and social privilege mediate the meaning of home, work, and women's labor. Hence, one can no longer assume that all women wanted the same opportunities in a conventionally defined wage labor market of work outside the home. The status and satisfaction that many women found as housewives, for example, can now be assessed relative to the drudgery they experienced as factory hands, mill workers, or domestic servants.[2] Wage work, housework, care work, and community work, as Alice Kessler-Harris reminds us, remain dynamic notions con-

---

[1] For an excellent historiographic review, see Eileen Boris and S. J. Kleinberg, "Mothers and Other Workers: (Re)Conceiving Labor, Maternalism, and the State," *Journal of Women's History* 15, no. 3 (2003): 90–117. See also Alice Kessler Harris, *In Pursuit of Equity: Women, Men and the Quest for Economic Citizenship in Twen-tieth Century America* (New York: Oxford University Press, 2001).

[2] See, for example, Judy Giles, "A Home of One's Own: Women and Domesticity in England, 1918–1950," *Women's Studies International Forum* 16 (1993): 239–53, and Sharon Harley, "For the Good of Family and Race: Gender, Work, and Domestic Roles in the Black Community, 1880–1930," *Signs* 15 (1990): 336–49.

stantly interpreted by those who actually balance all their competing demands.[3] Trained nursing initially offered white women a more authoritative public role. It eventually offered African American women a historically elusive goal of returning to more private roles to raise their own rather than other women's children.

But *American Nursing* also positions identity as well as paid and unpaid work at the center of its analysis. It engages with theoretical work that posits gender and gendered identities as sometimes situational and dependent on the context in which they are expressed and at other times serial and reflective of a sense of identification with several different groups. This approach allows me to more seriously consider nurses' perspectives about the meaning of their own claims to knowledge and expertise. It opens self-definition as a serious construct to be analyzed in its own right as well as in relation to the personal and political negotiations necessary in changing contexts. It also allows me to more fully consider how the interlocking concepts of race, class, and place, as well as gender, shape identity and knowledge claims. To this end, I am interested in the ways in which these concepts are embedded in all aspects of the history of American nursing, including the construction of knowledge about nursing practice, in the meaning of practice, and in the language and debates about how nurses understood and employed the meaning of professionalism.

Parts of the story I tell are transnational. In the early twentieth century, American nurses joined counterparts in Great Britain, Australia, Germany, and Canada in articulating an ideological foundation for the professionalism of their education and practice and in transforming the health and illness care delivered to millions across the globe. But nursing is, has been, and always will be a very private and intimate act performed in a particular place with its own imperatives, community norms, and local values. I am intrigued by the juxtaposition of what ideas about nursing, nurses, and care work transcend nation-state boundaries and what remain embedded in the context of place. I bring this perspective to my book. As my story unfolds, I also explore how gender, class, race, and place combine and come apart in different ways across a wide

[3] Alice Kessler-Harris, "Gender Ideology in Historical Reconstruction: A Case Study from 1930," *Gender and History* 1 (1989): 31–39.

range of temporal and social landscapes. I travel from the urban North to the rural South, from the perspectives of nursing educators to those of practicing clinicians, from lives lived as professionals to those lived as members of families and communities, from the dominant position of women nurses to the emerging one of men. I stop at places where issues of gender, class, and race coalesce in particular ways around nurses' identities, their claims to knowledge and expertise, and their relationships with each other, with those around them, and with their broader worlds.

These particular perspectives shape my book's main points. Individuals chose nursing, I argue, not only because of the work but also because of the meaning and power that a nursing identity brought to lives within families and local communities—both at particular moments and over the course of a lifetime. These women traded their work as students on the wards of hospitals throughout the United States for the expert knowledge, the specialized skills, and the additional education that promised to substantively broaden their range of choices in how they lived out their lives. This trade of work for knowledge did not always deliver on its promise of life as a nurse. Women left nursing over issues of too many nurses for too few positions, poor salaries, discriminatory employment practices, and the sometimes back-breaking labor involved in caring for the sick. But their sense of themselves as nurses—as competent and at times courageous women in control of at least parts of their own destiny—did open other possibilities as they recreated meaningful lives inside or outside nursing.

The chapters in this book develop the pieces of this argument chronologically and thematically. Chapter 1 looks to the experiences of lay and medical men and women as I reconstruct a narrative about the origins of modern trained nursing in nineteenth-century America. It looks specifically at the writings of mid- to later nineteenth-century Philadelphians, both men and women, who supported the medical education of women as physicians, as nurses, and as mothers. Philadelphia's experience was similar to those in its sister east coast cities of Boston and New York. But Philadelphia provides a particularly intriguing and exceptionally well-documented example of what was, in fact, a white, urban, middle-class knowledge project. Modern trained nursing, I argue, was born in the mutually constitutive process of women seeking knowledge and physicians seeking knowledgeable women. This was not the kind of knowledge emphasized by Florence Nightingale. Nightingale's emphasis on sanitary knowledge as that shared by all women, I argue, only reproduced the claims of class and social status of white middle-class mothers. By contrast, medical knowledge, drawn from the new tenets of science, taught by powerful physicians, and learned in a new hospital space, invited women who would train as nurses to invest themselves with an authority that would more effectively compete with maternal claims.

Chapter 2 moves to the later nineteenth and early twentieth centuries and explores how a small group of white, middle-class, female nursing leaders appropriated claims to control over particular elements of the nurses' training experience in their essays for lay audiences and their texts on nursing, professionalism, and ideal standards for training. This chapter takes seriously nurses' own emphasis on medical content and personal character. This emphasis certainly embodied the well-known traits of discipline, loyalty, and obedience. But such traits, I argue, also served in the production of even more important representations—or, in the words of one African American nurse, "impressions"—of competence, coolness, courage, and absolute control of clinical spaces. These representations created an internalized and fairly stable conceptualization of a strong nursing identity, albeit one shaded by the multiple meanings attached to nurses' particular gendered, racialized, and classed communities. Just as importantly, they allowed African American nurses, who identified with the same history and who survived the same formative processes of training, to appropriate and refashion a strong identity for the particular roles they played in their particular communities.

Chapter 3 describes the lives of nurses as identities forged in training confronted the realities of nursing's work. It compares the experiences of nurses on the West Coast, where the idea and the work of trained nurses were still novel, with those on the East Coast, where they had deeper roots. Nurses, I argue, were as powerful and resourceful as they were vulnerable and alienated. They protested the lack of sustained work—while seeking employment opportunities in other areas. They suffered through long, hard, and physically debilitating assignments—while saving and investing for some measure of financial independence. They endured returning to hospitals as paid staff—while waiting for more attractive positions to open in their operating rooms and out-patient departments. Their lives and their work existed at the fulcrum of race relations. Female African American nurses had more opportunities to learn and practice than African American male physicians. Yet their opportunities existed within the prerogatives of whiteness that took always took precedence over education and expertise.

Chapter 4 thinks more deeply and contextually about the meaning of identity and work among one group of white female nurses over the course of their lifetime. It focuses on the life stories of all the 1919 graduates of the Latter-Day Saints (LDS) Hospital Training School for Nurses in Salt Lake City, Utah. I make no claim that the experiences of the 1919 LDS Training School graduates were typical. But these stories provide a rare collective biography that allows me to explore the enor-mous range with which one group of white women—united only by reli-gion and a common training school experience—interpreted notions of what work meant over six decades of their lives. In these particular sto-ries, I argue, we see how a training school experience created a space for a one group of women to experience the promise of individual self-fulfillment and remain faithful to their church's pro-marriage, pro-family, and pronatalist teachings. This chapter also calls attention to the private, rather than public, strategies women used to navigate between personal aspirations and the demands of family life. I argue that the choice of nursing proved an effective strategy for those seeking to recon-cile conflicting desires, demands, and expectations in their personal and professional lives.

I travel south in chapter 5 to explore how the idea and the identity of trained nurses were not just willed and constructed but also contested. Georgia, and Atlanta in particular, provides a compelling site to con-sider the aspirations and the experiences of both white and African American women in a context where the idea of nursing strangers re-mained deeply embedded in overt social, sexualized, and racialized ste-reotypes. The experiences of nurses in Georgia show how both the idea and the identity of trained—or now registered—nurses depended, not just on women willing to do the work of nursing—on women willing to trade their work for meaningful, respected, and authoritative medical knowledge—but also on powerful social support for the women who would do such work.

Chapter 6 brings nurses out of their personal social communities and into those represented by state and national associations. I analyze nurses' own understanding of the meaning of "professionalism" as both an abstract construct and as a tool that—in some cases very reluctantly—helped nurses incorporate changing ideas and ideals into their social as well as professional identities. I look specifically at the post–World War II battle for the desegregation of the North Carolina State Nurses Association as emblematic of those occurring throughout the American south but as significant in that North Carolina is the only state with extant records that give voice to both the white and African American combatants. These data let me to examine carefully constructed discourses that allowed white and African American nurses to come together tentatively over an idea of professionalism in which shared class interests suppressed powerful racial divides.

I conclude by returning to the multiple meanings surrounding issues of women and work. Chapter 7 acknowledges a changed twenty-first-century context: the growth in the numbers of women working as physicians; the creation of new roles for nurses in advanced practice; and new benchmarks to mark the place of science, knowledge development, competence, and power in the discipline. But my concern in this chapter is to reframe the language and the politics of nursing to also include considerations of class, race, and community status. To this end, I compare data on the educational achievements of white, African American, Hispanic, and Asian nurses, not to physicians and other health care workers (which has been a more traditional point of comparison), but rather to women from their own race and ethnic communities. As we look ahead into the future of hospitals and health care, I argue, we continue to see how nurses trade work that transforms the care provided in American homes, hospitals, and health care systems for knowledge that changes their sense of themselves and their social place. But we also see, as the book draws to a close, how this trade works more powerfully for some women and men than it does for others.

I hope *American Nursing* continues a tradition in which the history of nurses and nursing becomes illustrative of broader themes in the history of women, medicine, work, and family. Susan Reverby in *Ordered to Care* and Darlene Clark Hine in *Black Women in White* have set the bar high. These histories have clearly illustrated the contextual limitations in nursing's historical quest for an independent role in hospitals and homes across the United States.[4]

My book, by contrast, is as concerned with the possibilities as with the problems. The nurses in my examples have different dreams and aspirations that may have only sometimes involved the actual work of nursing. But underpinning this heterogeneity is a phenomenon for which other disciplines now strive but which few have needed to achieve. Individuals from many different backgrounds have historically joined together around a sustained and deeply internalized disciplinary identity. As this history of nurses and nursing suggests, there are significant problems when this identity finds little validation in the wider world. But when one shifts the focus from work to the meaning of the work to lives in families, communities, and, for some, the broader national stage, one also sees some direction as nurses and nursing move into the twenty-first century. More explicitly integrating the language surrounding gender, class, race, and place will broaden the base of social and political support necessary to support nursing's tradition of caring for the sick and caring for practitioners as diverse as the patients they treat.

[4]Susan Reverby, *Ordered to Care: The Dilemma of American Nursing, 1850–1945* (New York: Cambridge University Press, 1987); Darlene Clark Hine, *Black Women in White: Racial Conflict and Cooperation in the Nursing Profession, 1890–1950* (Bloomington: Indiana University Press, 1989).

American Nursing

CHAPTER 1

Nurses and Physicians in Nineteenth-Century Philadelphia

I N 1886, the Board of Lady Managers of the Woman's Hospital of Phil-adelphia considered its twenty-five-year history. The hospital had opened in 1861 with an ambitious agenda: it would care for poor women, educate lay women about their own health and that of their families, and be the first American hospital to provide formal clinical experiences to women who would be physicians and nurses. The Woman's Hospital accomplished its mission. Over the succeeding decades, the hospital's former medical and nursing students had formed a web of skilled prac-titioners throughout the United States. Nurse Harriet Phillips, an 1869 graduate of the Woman's Hospital Training School, worked with Native Americans in Wisconsin before assuming the role of the first matron of the Chinese Mission Home, a refuge for destitute Chinese prostitutes established by San Francisco's Presbyterian women philanthropists in the 1870s.[1] Wealthy San Francisco women supported Dr. Charlotte Blake Brown when she returned to her native city in 1875 and began both a clinic for women and children and the first training school for nurses on the West Coast.[2] Meanwhile, the Mormon sister-wives Ellis Reynolds Shipp and Margaret Curtis Shipp helped each other through their 1870s Philadelphia medical training and clinical experiences at the Woman's Hospital. When they returned to their native Utah, they worked with the women's Relief Society of the Church of Jesus Christ of the Latter-day Saints to establish the formal School of Obstetrics and Nursing in Salt Lake City.[3]

Yet much had changed in twenty-five years. More and more women were gaining admission to coeducational medical schools. A small but growing number of large and prestigious hospitals were now using stu-dent nurses to care for their patients and to manage the day-to-day routine of the wards. The Woman's Hospital Board of Lady Managers took full credit for these medical and nursing accomplishments. In particular, their nurses training school graduates, they boasted, had already laid the groundwork for specialized education and skilled practice long before the better known and more widely publicized schools at Bellevue Hospital in New York City, the New Haven Hospital in Connecticut, and the Massachusetts General Hospital in Boston had even opened in the early 1870s. These three schools self-consciously linked their nurses training with the ideals of Florence Nightingale, the iconic and still active and opinionated "Lady with the Lamp." But, as the Lady Managers proudly wrote, it was Woman's Hospital nursing graduates who made these schools a reality. Amanda Judson, an 1871 training school graduate, was the head nurse of the Nightingale-styled training ward at Bellevue; and Emily Bayard, an 1872 graduate, had opened and led the Connecticut Training School at the New Haven Hospital.[4]

For the Board of Lady Managers, the success of women physicians and nurses was inexorably linked. "Not until the true status of women in medicine was recognized," they wrote in their 1886 annual report, "was the want fully met of a band of thoroughly trained nurses." Certainly, historians have also long recognized the ties that bound the nineteenth-century initiatives to provide for the formal clinical education, experience, and practice of women physicians and nurses in the northeastern urban centers of the United States. Both the New York Infirmary for Women and Children, opened in 1857, and the New England Hospital for Women and Children, opened in Boston in 1862, placed the training of nurses as central to their stated missions of women treating other women.[5]

In seeking to reconstruct a narrative about the origins of what we today consider professional nursing, this chapter explores the experiences among lay women like the Woman's Hospital managers, supportive medical colleagues, and nurses. It looks specifically at the mid- to late nineteenth-century experiences of several generations of lay and medical Philadelphia men and women who supported the medical education of women—as mothers, as nurses, and as physicians. It argues that the origins of modern trained nursing lay in the idea that it would engage particular women with valued, valuable, and even exciting medical knowledge that conferred a specific form of socially appropriate and legitimate

authority. This was not just the sanitary knowledge of an earlier generation and emphasized by Nightingale. This was also knowledge about
how to make scientific sense of vigilant clinical observations that determined how treatment might proceed. And, notwithstanding Nightingale's strident assertion that nurses were not "medical women," this
chapter argues, to reiterate the point made in the introduction, that
modern nursing was born in the mutually constitutive process of women
seeking medical knowledge and physicians seeking knowledgeable
women.

Nursing the Sick

The work of sick nursing in mid-nineteenth-century Philadelphia—the
day-in, day-out work of cleaning, bathing, turning, feeding, administering medications, and preparing nutritious foods—took place at home.
Home, irrespective of one's place in the class, ethnic, and racial ordering
of the city, still represented the best, safest, and most comforting site for
treatment and care as well as for birthing and dying. The work of sick
nursing was messy, chaotic, and unpredictable as moments of crises
followed hours of monotony. It required intimate body work: it meant
cleaning the sweat, blood, vomit, urine, and feces as some patients were
wasting from fevers and as others were responding to treatments.[6] And
it required skilled body work—skills often learned only at the moment
they were needed, but skills upon which a patient's recovery depended.
For example, sick nurses needed to know how to apply blisters and care
for the irritated skin after such applications, how to prepare different
kinds of poultices, and how to administer enemas or douches. They also
needed to bring judgment and insight to their work; they needed to bring
less tangible skills sometimes described as just plain "common sense"
and at other times praised as those of careful discrimination and observation. They needed to be able to read a patient's body and stop a particular treatment at that finely calibrated moment when it had had its
desired effect but had not become the cause of a patient's worsening
condition.

Sick nursing also demanded intense monitoring of one's own emotions. It meant dampening fears of contagion and feelings of disgust that
came with such close body work. It also meant tolerating the frustration

that often attended the labile moods of patients. This emotional work of sick nursing could be as intense as it was intimate. As historian Emily Abel has argued, it often took place within a matrix of family relationships shaped as much by resentments and inescapable responsibilities as by affection and deliberate choice.[7]

Nursing often seemed like an intensely private and even isolating experience. But the site of the work—the sick room—could be a very public place. A critical part of the work of sick nursing, in fact, involved mediating between such private and public spaces. Nurses had to monitor the physical boundaries between the sick room and the wider world. They had to attend, for example, to the cleanliness and ventilation of the sick room and to the movement of objects such as diet trays and linens into and out of the room in a quiet and orderly manner. They also had to tame the inevitable tendency toward chaos in the sick room. As the instructions of one patient laid out so clearly in 1845, sick nurses had to ensure that one person—not necessarily herself but perhaps a friend or a servant—would "take the lead and see everything is done the way it should be done, when it should be done, and that this consistency is carried through day-in-and-day out."[8] And they had to attend to the social boundaries: they had to ensure peace and quiet, eliminate what another commentator felt to be the "particularly annoying" tendency of others to whisper outside the closed door, and, if necessary, refuse the admission of those who might be intrusive, upsetting, or too full of their own advice and opinions.[9]

Defining Sick Nursing

If the actual work of sick nursing remained recognizable and relatively easily described, the meaning of that work was, by contrast, malleable and remarkably fluid. Nursing was gendered and racialized: images of ideal sick nurses oscillated between devoted white, middle-class mothers and faithful, perhaps enslaved African American "mammies." But not all sick nurses were women. Inebriated or insane men, epidemics, natural disasters, dangerous injuries, and the simple unavailability of anyone else also required the assistance of fathers, husbands, brothers, and neighbors.[10]

Sick nursing also meant negotiating the often unstable nature of the power relationships inherent in the day-to-day interactions about the work. Ideally, sick nurses would perform a complicated calculus among competing interests when considering how to care for their patients. They would consider the physicians' directives, their own judgment, and their patient's wishes.[11] In the free-wheeling, entrepreneurial, and competitive world of nineteenth-century medicine, the physician might be a Thomsonian herbalist prescribing a course of lobelia, a homeopath recommending a series of "infinitesimal" preparations, or a medical doctor titrating the proper dose of an opiate to relieve pain. But as historians have pointed out, all mid-century physicians' claims of knowledge and expertise directly confronted and often collided with those of sick nurses and their patients.[12] Indeed, Andrew Todd Thomson, a British physician whose domestic nursing manual had been republished in Philadelphia in 1845, remarked in horror about an ill colleague who rejected every prescription proposed by his medical friends. He placed his confidence instead in a "nostrum" proffered by—of all people—the wife of his coachman.[13] This colleague suffered a proper and prescriptive end: he died.

Despite such warnings, sick nurses believed in the usefulness of knowledge learned in public health and hygiene lectures as well as in domestic medicine and nursing texts. They also valued the generations of wisdom passed on through families' familiar receipt books and folk wisdom. And they respected the experience and expertise of other nurses. For example, in her 1837 *Family Nurse*, the companion book to her widely popular *The Frugal Housewife*, Lydia Child assured her readers that her suggestions about caring for the sick had been reviewed and approved by an eminent physician. But her authority drew as well, she continued, from her own experiences, the advice of her aged relatives, and those whom she had found to be "judicious" nurses.[14]

But Child's authority never matched that of Florence Nightingale. The U.S. edition of Nightingale's *Notes on Nursing: What It Is and What It Is Not* appeared in 1860. The reception was overwhelming. *Godey's Lady's Book* hailed it as a "monument to the power of truth" and as "one of the most important books ever put forth by women."[15] *Quarterly Review* called it nothing less than "a work of genius."[16] Philadelphia's own

Saturday Evening Post took advantage of lax copyright laws and, between March and May 1860, serialized the entire book in special weekly sections.

Notes on Nursing presented little new knowledge about how to care for either the well or the sick. Its popularity and persuasiveness drew from Nightingale's celebrated experiences as a nurse in England's Crimean War and as an educated woman deeply concerned about women's control over women's domain. Nightingale's idealized sick nurse was a thinking and thoughtful mother, capable of making independent judgments and of assessing the medical qualifications of those physicians who entered her domain. Nightingale reserved her strongest contempt for women who refused to assume these responsibilities. "Did nature," she sarcastically wondered about those who fled to physicians for advice about nursing, "always intend mothers to be accompanied by doctors?"[17] She was just as scornful of those who blindly followed the advice of "fashionable" doctors who offered the kinds of remedies that, in her opinion, treated only the whims and fancies of their clientele. Rather, she strongly supported the practices of those she called "thinking physicians": well-educated men who had studied at leading medical schools and who called upon years of careful "observation and experience" when approaching their sick patients.[18]

Nightingale's nurse was a disciplined and completely committed administrator (if not something of a martinet) "in charge" of one's home and one's help, doing what she needed to do, and making sure that everyone else was doing the assigned tasks as well.[19] Gender was critical. Nightingale could no more understand why gifted women might wish to doctor than Elizabeth Blackwell, her famous physician friend and correspondent, could understand why they might want to nurse.[20] For Nightingale, the gendered nature of nursing allowed it to transcend social place. It joined all women in shared knowledge even as it solidified the gender boundaries between their practices and those of physicians. Nursing knowledge was distinct from medical knowledge: it was "everyday sanitary knowledge" of fresh air, warmth, proper ventilation, nutritious diets, exemplary hygiene, and calm environments that all women—be they ladies, servants, or what Nightingale called "professional" nurses—needed to assume responsibility for learning and for wielding.[21] Yet a nurse's white, middle-class, maternal martinet status was assumed. *Notes on Nursing* specifically spoke to women who would supervise staff who performed the body work of sick nursing. Her later *Notes on Nursing for the Labouring Classes,* published in London in 1861 and never reviewed in American middle-class magazines, had a different focus. Nightingale never condescended to the working-class audience for which *Notes on Nursing for the Labouring Classes* was intended. The content of the "sanitary knowledge" she wished to spread remained the same. This book, however, had a different ending. *Notes on Nursing* cautioned readers not to interfere with the work of the "professional nurse" in their homes. *Notes on Nursing for the Labouring Classes,* by contrast, ended with specific directions about the body work of sick nursing that these very different readers would perform for their own or for others' families.[22]

The Context of Care

Nineteenth-century sick nursing existed at the uneasy intersection of class interests, knowledge, and identities. In Philadelphia's increasingly commercialized economy, a place where work itself had become a commodity to be bought or sold in the wage labor market, the ability to hire (or, conversely, to be hired as) a sick nurse represented one of many activities that served to shape an emerging divide between the white working class and the middle class in the mid-nineteenth-century city.[23] Physician commentators on nursing, assuming the invisibility of race, focused on these class distinctions between nursing women. They drew careful distinctions between the judgment and the intellect that properly "educated" middle-class mothers brought to the sick nursing of their families and the "prejudices" and "superstitions" that shaped the practices of servants and working-class hired nurses.[24]

The idea of hired nurses—of paying for nursing—raised profound ambivalence. Hired nurses certainly provided much-needed assistance during periods of acute illnesses. It was yet another mark of middle-class status and economic security. Paying for nursing also served as a testament to a community's responsibility for, and ability to help, its own sick poor. This was a particular point of pride for Philadelphia's African American community. In an 1831 advertisement in the *Philadelphia Gazette,* this community strongly protested the state's pending legislation to limit the rights of both enslaved African Americans who sought refuge in the city and those of free African Americans who already lived there. This advertisement pointed with pride to more than forty-three voluntary associations run by African American men and women throughout the city that had provided more than $6,000 to their own sick and destitute. They served as proof, the advertisement continued, that the African American community had as strong a sense of civic responsibility as any other and that it was not only willing but also able to save its sick and destitute from the humiliation of needing public assistance.[25]

But however necessary, valuable, and fulfilling such assistance might be, actually needing the care of hired nurses meant risking one's own vulnerability to strangers who, in other circumstances, one might master, or to whom one might minister. This vulnerability had often stoked the fires of simmering anxiety and sometimes frank resentment toward those who would accept positions as hired nurses. White Philadelphians, for example, needed the help of the free African American community during the 1793 yellow fever epidemic. But such a need went hand in hand with anger and a sense of exploitation that many white Philadelphians felt about the high wages these men and women commanded. White Philadelphians often devalued the care provided by free African Americans during the epidemic. As Jacqueline Miller argues, however, this devaluation was less a reflection of the skill of their actual work than a focus of anxiety about the destabilizing threat of their high wages to the carefully classed and raced labor market.[26] It was an effort to justify a return to much lower wages.

Needing the care of paid nurses also inverted the well-understood and reciprocal rituals of obligation and deference that normally surrounded the work of white working- and middle-class women. The drunk and callous nurses "Sairey Gamp" and "Betsy Prigg" created by Charles Dickens in his 1844 book *Martin Chuzzlewit* ignored their patients to the horror of an audience imagining themselves in similar situations. Although, as historian Anne Summers has argued, most working-class hired nurses were likely more unrefined than unkind and uncaring, anxieties and resentments about hired nurses persisted through the Civil War.[27] The most reassuring message one might send to a family about a loved one's final hours was that, as their soldier lay dying, no "hired hand" had ever touched his body.[28]

Most of Philadelphia's mid-nineteenth-century paid nurses left few traces. Lisa Rosner's reconstruction of Philadelphia's early nineteenth-century medical marketplace mirrors Susan Reverby's analysis of one group of mid-century nurses who turned for assistance in their old age to Boston's Home for Aged Women. Both suggest that hired nurses tended to enter the market at ages older than other women workers, usually pushed there by the poverty and destitution that so often accompanied the widowhood, divorce, or abandonment of nineteenth-century working-class women.[29] Certainly, for some men and women, sick nursing was a way to a craft identity in the wage labor market. But for most, it was not the sole source of identity. The advertisements in mid-nineteenth-century American newspapers placed by those seeking full-time live-in work, for example, spoke to the multiple skills that some women offered to the domestic labor market. They offered skills as both a housekeeper and a nurse, as both a cook and a nurse, as both a chambermaid and a nurse.[30] One advertisement sought to sell a slave: this woman was certainly a "good cook and washer," but more importantly, she was also "an excellent nurse."[31]

For most women and some men, then, sick nursing represented a moment in lives filled with other responsibilities. Nursing the sick was an acknowledged part, but only a part, of lives lived as parents, spouses, siblings, friends, neighbors, and workers. Sometimes it was a long moment. In Jane Schultz's reconstruction of Civil War nursing, some 20,000 women from different classes and races and from both the North and the South formally volunteered, were hired by their respective governments, or, as did Clara Barton, simply showed up to work as nurses. Most worked alone or with one or two other women. But when in larger encampments, those few privileged women who could afford to volunteer their nursing work kept themselves carefully apart—ideologically and socially—from those who worked for wages. In addition, nurses maintained careful class and race boundaries around discrete categories of nursing work. Nurses and matrons were disproportionately white; cooks and laundresses, who did the hardest and least skilled labor, were disproportionately African American.[32]

Not surprisingly, such categories often collapsed in the press of day-to-day experiences and demands. Catholic nuns, a small but visible number of Civil War nurses, were renowned for their willingness to do whatever needed to be done without distinction and without complaint. But free African Americans often needed to assert their privilege over former slaves. And tensions flared when white, middle-class women were asked to perform what they saw as menial labor unconnected to the direct care of soldiers. Their response replicated the power relationships of their lives at home: they simply hired their presumed social subordinates—working-class women or African American women—to mop blood-drenched floors, wash clothes soaked with mud and gore, empty slop buckets, or mend torn clothing. And when the war was over, these women's moment of nursing was over. They returned home and reconstructed lives that, even when they needed to work, did not involve the work of hired nursing.[33]

The Needs of Thinking Physicians

The women who served as nurses during the Civil War returned home to the nineteenth century's continuing medical mantra among the "thinking physicians" whom Nightingale admired: The best efforts of a physician, it constantly reiterated, were for naught without the work of careful and skilled nurses. These "thinking"—or, as historian John Harley Warner has characterized them, "intellectually active"—physicians shared a common social background among the middling and upper classes of their communities. They also shared a rigorous form of medical education. They first attended lectures by distinguished American physicians in prominent medical schools connected, however loosely, with leading universities. They then often secured prestigious house staff positions at the few American hospitals that provided clinical experiences. And they frequently studied abroad at the leading European medical centers in France and, after the Civil War, in Germany.[34]

Philadelphia had, in fact, already been the site of several significant, albeit unsuccessful, attempts by such "thinking physicians" to teach women the specific skills they felt were necessary to nurse sick patients. In 1839 Joseph Warrington, a graduate of the University of Pennsylvania Medical College, one of the most prestigious medical schools in the country, had started the Nurse Society of Philadelphia to train white working-class women to serve as educated assistants to physicians during childbirth.[35] Supported by "intelligent and liberal minded ladies," he envisioned nurses who, like the midwives they would replace, would still be available to care for other women in childbirth but would, unlike the midwives, be trained by a physician and responsible to him rather than to the parturient woman. His *Nurses Guide,* a text for both these nurses and the birthing women they would assist, was ambitious. It was full of explicit medical language, rationales for scientific treatments, and precise descriptions of physiological events that marked signs of healing or symptoms of impending crises. The *Nurses Guide* hoped to construct an idea of a new kind of nurse who, in the ideologically and economically competitive medical marketplace, would support a particular physician's knowledge claims and practice because she understood and participated in the careful science upon which it built. But it also reinforced traditional knowledge, gender, and class hierarchies. The formal education and training that such physicians might deny midwives, they would give to nurses: to nursing wives and mothers for a more informed supervisory place within their family; to hired nurses in exchange for education, opportunity, and greater authority within the hierarchy of the household's domestic staff; and to all for partnership in support of a particular kind of doctoring that would be now characterized, as Warrington wrote, by "mutual confidence."[36]

This idea of trading of medical knowledge for responsible, respectable, and authoritative nursing work failed to attract many working-class women. The numbers of middle-class women wanting to hire working-class women trained by the Nurse Society always exceeded the supply.[37] Still, in 1842, Joseph Longshore, another Philadelphia physician and graduate of the University of Pennsylvania Medical College tried again— but now outside the lying-in chamber. He published *The Principles and Practice of Nursing* or, as its title went on to explain, *A Guide to the Inexperience*—be they families, nurses, or young physicians. *Principles and Practices,* he cautioned, would not concentrate on "detail of minutiae" about what a nurse should do: only the physician would make such decisions. Rather, the book would concentrate on "general physiological principles" and the application of such knowledge to the care of those suffering from what he called general diseases.[38] Book sales were a source of keen disappointment.[39]

In fact, the trade of medical knowledge for authoritative work proposed by both Warrington and Longshore was founded on the assumed superiority of a particular kind of knowledge that, in mid-nineteenth-century Philadelphia, was still contested. Moreover, the trade reflected the somewhat presumptuous belief that an invitation to participate in their world of science, learning, and propriety as a servant might grant a working-class woman more status than that conferred by her reputation and nursing practice within her own community of friends and family. In fact, the proffered trade only reinforced class boundaries. Even as Warrington and Longshore were hoping to train working-class women as nurses, they were simultaneously training women from their own social background to become physicians.

Women Physicians and "Responsible" Nurses

Women physicians were as interested as were their male colleagues in teaching all women how to nurse. Ann Preston, Warrington and Longshore's most successful medical protégé, once again attempted to tease out all the conflicting claims of class, knowledge, and authority in her 1863 book *Nursing the Sick and the Training of Nurses*.[40] Preston was part of Philadelphia's small group of activists committed to the formal education of women as traditionally trained medical practitioners. She had studied with Warrington, was among the first graduates as well as the first female dean of the Female Medical College of Pennsylvania, and had worked closely with the women philanthropists who had established the Woman's Hospital of Philadelphia in 1861.[41]

But Preston and her women colleagues continuously struggled with the gendered orthodoxy of their practice.[42] Even supporters of women physicians had reservations about the appropriateness of their practicing all aspects of medicine. Certainly, one magazine editorial stated, if a woman were to enter any of the professions, medicine would be the one particularly attractive to both her "tastes and habits" and to her innate commitment to the care of the sick and the relief of human suffering. Still, it continued, "we are not convinced, and do not believe, that the *highest* departments of medicine . . . [that involve] the most difficult and obstinate cases [and] especially such as require surgical treatment" fall within women's domain. These cases demanded more than medical knowledge obtained from books; they demanded "long experience, and the firmness, the nerve, and even the physical strength of a man."[43]

Women physicians were well aware of these tensions. Longshore, one of their first supporters, seemed to have little interest in exactly what women might do with formal medical knowledge. However sincere his interest in training women as physicians, his biographer noted, he came to it only after so few responded to his call to nursing. Moreover, their experiences as students at the Female Medical College had already raised concerns that they were being prepared to be something less than "full doctors." Their male teachers, they complained, had rather decided ideas that as women they would practice as excellent and educated consultants, midwives, and nurses within the circumscribed worlds of lying-in chambers, nurseries, and women's hospitals.[44]

Preston, in response, clearly differentiated her role from that of other women. She forthrightly asserted the credibility of her place, her voice, and her authority as a medical expert—not only on the health and illness care of women and children but also on nursing. Certainly, she wrote in *Nursing the Sick*, all women did not share the same social standing. But all women needed the same knowledge about the care of the sick. In fact, in the formal nurses training school at the Woman's Hospital, women who nursed families and those who nursed the hospital's patients received the same lectures from the same physicians as they sat side by side in the hospital's classroom. The "ladies," as they were called, paid two dollars for a course of ten lectures on nursing, but those "responsible nurses expecting to follow that occupation" paid only seventy-five cents. Apart from sporadic supervision on the wards, there was little specific content that differentiated the instruction of mothers from that of Preston's nurses.[45]

Preston's "responsible" nurses would not be mothers (in her mind God's best nurses), and they could not be nuns (her second-best nurses, particularly fitted for public roles in hospitals). But they would come close. Preston called those who would train as nurses "novitiates," a term that linked them to the aspiration of those who would take religious vows. She hoped to fashion a role where they acted in the temporary place of mothers, but their strength would be that they were not mothers.

"Families worn down with the long and extreme illness of a member require relief," she reminded her audience. "And a stranger whose feelings will be less intensely taxed, and who can therefore better endure the labor, for a time, is desirable."[46]

Knowledge might be shared in this gendered world of women physicians and nurses. Power would not. Preston, in ways that echoed Nightingale, outlined clear differences in the class roles between those who would nurse their own families and those who would do so among strangers in others' homes or in hospitals. Middle-class women certainly needed to know how to nurse. They needed to have an "appreciation of the importance of familiarity with those practical details which will make them invaluable in sickness and sorrow." But they did not have to do all of it. They could, if they so chose, hire capable assistants. These assistants would consider their nursing as a "business" and would help, in particular, with the body work of nursing—with the bathing, turning, cooking for, and cleaning that all sick patients needed. This realignment of roles resonated perfectly with white, middle-class expectations. Middle-class women were already managing the servants and the cooks working inside their homes—men and women trading work for money in an increasingly commercialized economy. Preston now asked that they know enough to supervise the sick nurses they would hire. And she asked her readers to join with physicians and seek out suitable women and encourage them to consider nursing as a business.[47]

But Preston's recruitment strategy to the Woman's Hospital Nurses Training School failed miserably. The numbers of nurses in training rarely exceeded one or two during the 1860s. For nursing care, the hospital depended on persons recruited by direct advertisement, convalescing patients with the strength to care for others, and medical students. The women who would be nurses stayed away. There seemed little reason to drop their own claims to experience and accede to that which was privileged by class rather than expertise. The mid-century process of sick nursing remained more about who one was—a mother, a nun, or a hired assistant—than about what one knew or what one did. To practice it in the home for love was to reify one's maternal identity. To practice it in exchange for wages with strangers kept one within the servant sphere. Preston recognized this inherent contradiction. Privately and pragmatically, she and the Woman's Hospital's Board of Lady Managers hoped that the possibility of training nurses might allow the hospital to "do away with the necessity for the service of chamber maids."[48]

A Changing World of Science and Scientific Practice

Traditionally trained and "thinking" physicians had long been committed to differentiating themselves and their practice from all other traditions of nineteenth-century healing. They held a vision of themselves as participating in a learned and scientific profession worthy of confidence in its acts of healing. Central to its acts of healing—the knowledge that would set their practice apart from and above the claims of other kinds of medical practitioners—was the manipulation of carefully selected therapeutic agents, treatments, and hygienic practices that would actively—and, if necessary, heroically—rescue patients from their diseases.[49] Certainly, knowledge about anatomy, physiology, and chemistry had long been critical to understanding therapeutic principles. But in postbellum America, a small group of influential and ambitious traditionally trained physicians—as well as their informed lay supporters—increasingly placed their faith in the new ideas about science and scientific practice.

These new ideas involved an emphasis on laboratory science that would now focus on seemingly objective physiological processes and chemical analyses. They included practices that would depend upon the quantification of clinical signs and symptoms—on the careful and graphic representations of temperatures, pulses, and respiration rates—to determine the course and effectiveness of prescribed treatments. They placed less significance on the subjective, idiosyncratic, and personalized descriptions of families and patients. Just as importantly, they depended upon a recalculation of competing interests—one in which sick nurses would attach greater weight to physicians' directives than to their patients' wishes or to their own judgments. Charles Putman, speaking before the American Social Science Association in 1874 as a physician seeking broader social support for the formal training of nurses, directly connected the rise of medicine as a science with that of nursing. "If we desire to make a science of our art," he told his audience, to know if, and exactly how much, and after what time, and in what respect, our digitalis effects the pulse, and our calomel the temperature, or the daily or hourly variations in pulse and temperature from any cause, or if we wish to know the character of the excretions throughout the day, or to test the doctrine of crisis in our practice; or if we wish to give cold baths of a definite temperature in typhoid fever, or to have the ear syringed out so that the fluid will go where it is wanted, or leeches or cups applied, or subcutaneous injections given, we cannot do it without the aid of skilled nurses.[50]

These new ideas about science and scientific practice slowly transformed the place of the hospital in the medical armamentarium. The hospital had always reflected traditions of pious activism, stewardship, and class. It embodied the reciprocal responsibility of the blessed toward the poor without family or friends to care for them in times of illness. One would give, and the other would remain worthy of and grateful for receipt of, such care. The nineteenth-century hospital also had long recognized its responsibility to support the education and practice of traditionally trained physicians. But now such physicians also saw it as a site that could produce even newer scientific knowledge. Northern Civil War hospitals had already been praised for their ability to create new procedures that staved off the infections that seemed the almost inevitable fate of those on crowded wards or in complicated surgeries, and good nursing was acknowledged as central to this achievement. The hope was now that these triumphs, and particularly the surgical triumphs, might be pushed even further. And the task remained that of training good nurses.[51]

Samuel Gross, an eminent Civil War surgeon and professor at Jefferson Medical College in Philadelphia, took up this challenge. There was little new and even less that was controversial in his 1869 report to the American Medical Association, an organization founded in 1847 by traditionally trained physicians in support of their particular practice. Fresh from fame in the Civil War's hospitals, Gross praised the potential of both hospitals and military hierarchies in which physicians and nurses worked. But there were now careful changes in language and emphasis. Certainly, he noted, "the commander of an army cannot be victorious if he is not properly aided by his subordinate lieutenants." The physician was the commander, and the nurses were the lieutenants. But the analogy of the trained nurse as lieutenant also implied a significant amount of power. Granted, Gross conceded, her primary responsibility was to carry out orders. But within the hospital or the sickroom at home, the trained nurse, like an army's lieutenant, would also have the power to independently attend to the "minor details" that might distract the physician commander. She would also have the knowledge and the training, again like her military counterpart, to take effective and immediate charge in the chaotic moments of the unexpected crises and emergencies that occurred in the absence of the physician commander.[52]

This trained nurse would be equally powerful outside the sickroom. As one carefully trained by and aligned with one group of physicians committed to the legitimacy of their own practice, she could subvert the practices of other physicians. In particular, she would have the knowledge to judge the quality of the medical treatment given to her patient. And she would have the authority to step outside traditional hierarchies of deference—be they classed or gendered—and challenge a particular practitioner and practice that seemed to threaten a patient's recovery. The properly trained nurse, Gross quite frankly reminded his audience, could "do much to correct the errors of an ignorant, careless, or unscrupulous physician."[53]

But creating this new nurse meant supplanting other nurses. Certainly, Gross played out the usual castigation of paid nurses in home and public hospitals. But he also now turned on mothers and daughters. Gross was well aware that he was criticizing what he admitted were the ninety-nine out of a hundred nurses caring for their sick families at home. But these mothers and daughters were "wholly unfit." They assumed responsibility for nursing their families while blissfully and "totally ignorant of the first principles of nursing."[54]

Gross was not alone in this new and harsh critique of women nursing their families at home. In 1872, S. Weir Mitchell, a Philadelphia physician and national expert on nervous diseases of women, spoke just as bluntly to wives and mothers in *Lippincott's Magazine of Popular Literature and Science*. The only role for physicians in most instances of sickness within families, in his mind, was to place themselves firmly between the patients and their mothers. Physicians had to save their patients from the dosing and the over-dosing of their mothers and allow the therapy of time to work its cure. Moreover, in times of critical illnesses, mothers created an environment of "fuss and disorder" when the patient, in fact, needed "the cool control, calm and steady discipline that only a stranger can provide." Mothers were "amateurs," and he admitted his astonishment that Nightingale said so little about this kind of nursing in her classic book.[55]

The critique continued. Abram Livezy, a widely cited medical authority on the health of children, railed against mothers in *Peterson's Magazine,* another popular woman's publication. In his "Mothers' Department," a regularly occurring column that ran through the 1870s, he branded the fashion of self-prescribing or of following the advice of friends and family as "mischievous and reprehensible" and said that tampering with those medications prescribed by physicians was "dangerous, to say the least."[56] And still later, the physician Frank Fisher, writing in *The Ladies' Home Journal and Practical Housekeeper* in 1889, cautioned his readers against assuming that they—and they alone—knew how to nurse their families. They did not: their judgment, he warned them, "has been warped . . . by affectionate anxiety." The result was that every little cough or sigh or change in temperament became an immediate medical crisis, and the physician would be unnecessarily called to the bedside.[57]

"Thinking Nurses"

This devaluing of personalized maternal knowledge, experiences, and trustworthiness went hand in hand with prominent physicians' ideas about the demands of scientific practice and research. James Hinton, a British physician whose popular *Thoughts on Health* had been serialized in Philadelphia magazines in the 1870s, argued that medical science needed trained nurses since there now existed "fresh methods of investigation so numerous, so exact and complex, and demanding for their proper application so much time" that they demanded the scientific work that could only be done by a trained and true nurse. This nurse would simultaneously benefit the patient in her care and, just as importantly, "provide materials on which the future life of medicine might base itself."[58] The American physician William Thompson echoed these sentiments. When reporting on the slowly increasing numbers of formal nurses' training schools in 1888, he acknowledged the place of training in offering women more options for economic self-support. But the primary benefit, he argued, accrued to medicine and to medical knowledge. As physicians sought to advance their science, he wrote, they needed "intelligent and conscientious nurses" who would fulfill their orders to the letter and who could be trusted to observe, record, and if necessary act immediately upon the variations of signs and symptoms presented by their patients' responses to prescribed therapeutics.[59] "Thinking physicians" needed thinking nurses.

These "thinking nurses" still required Nightingale's sanitary knowledge. In fact, as other historians have pointed out, the careful management of diet, rest, fresh air, exercise, and cleanliness remained central to later nineteenth-century medical and nursing practice, at homes and in hospitals, by mothers and by hired nurses.[60] But intellectually ambitious physicians now spoke of "scientific nursing" as an adjunct to and, when necessary, as a temporary surrogate for "scientific doctoring."[61] Scientific nursing was a process of understanding the anatomical, physiological, chemical, and bacteriological rationales for what was to be done and, just as importantly, why it was to be done in a particular way. It was, as reinterpreted by nurse Clara Weeks, a process of "nursing by reason rather than by rule."[62] It depended on the manipulation of new technologies such as the thermometer, and on the completion of new procedures such as urine analyses, which would provide the almost hour-by-hour data that guided healing and care work; it depended, in nurse Elizabeth Gregg's perspective, on the "patient, painstaking" attention to the details that ultimately revealed the causes of disease.[63] As James Wilson, a member of Philadelphia's prestigious College of Physicians and visiting physician at two prominent Philadelphia hospitals, wrote in *Fever Nursing* in 1888, the healing work of physicians and trained nurses had to be "interdependent." But, he continued, the physician's work also depended on the presence of a nurse capable of "independent thought and action" during the sudden changes in conditions or in the emergencies that inevitably occurred during the course of a patients' illness.[64]

Many lay commentators agreed. As one of them noted of his own family's experiences, it was the trained nurse's skill, her commitment to carrying out the physician's orders with "utmost fidelity," and her vigilant observations and careful recordings of temperature, pulse, and respirations that helped save his critically ill son's life. The "utmost accuracy" of her work, he believed, allowed the physician to judge the effects of treatment and the progress of the disease.[65] Some commentators protested such attempts to replace traditional maternal duties and scorned such mothers who would participate. "These luxurious times," one person wrote in 1893, "find mothers so oppressed with social duties, so absorbed in reading and writing and calling and entertaining, in dressing and in planning dresses, so dependent on servants, that, what are, after all, important accomplishments like knowing how to be a family nurse have been allowed to become out-of-date."[66] But another wrote that a mother's "affection, however warm, will not qualify a sick-nurse." Instead, the "cool head and steady hand of a professional stranger is too often to be preferred."[67]

The Idea and the Reality

Turning the idea of scientific nursing into reality, however, was tortuous and slow—every bit as slow as that of turning the age-old process of doctoring into its new vision of scientific medicine. Not all elite physicians saw medicine's future in the epistemological preciseness of the laboratory, the fever graphs, and the careful charting of a treatment's effect.[68] And not all believed that the key to this future lay with trained nurses. Even the most supportive of physicians needed reassurances that the practice of trained nursing would not bleed into that of doctoring. Horatio Storer, a strong physician believer in the importance of formal nurses training, admitted the pervasive concern "that the nurse, by endeavoring to advance, might exceed her sphere; and that in attempting to do better she would do more."[69]

Nightingale practically shrieked her reassurances from across the Atlantic. "You say," she wrote back to a physician considering the possibility of a new training school at Bellevue Hospital in New York City in 1872, that "the great difficulty will be to define the instructions, the duties, and the position of the nurses" as distinct from those of physicians. "Is this a difficulty?" she responded with her underlined emphasis.

A nurse is not a "medical man" nor is she a medical woman. Most carefully do we avoid in our training the confusion, both practically and theoretically, of letting women suppose that nursing duties and medical duties run into or overlap each other—so much so that, though we have often been asked to allow ladies intending to be "Doctors" to come in as *Nurses* to St. Thomas' Hospital, in order to "pick up," so they phrased it, "professional medical knowledge," we have never consented even to admit such applicants to avoid even the semblance of encouraging such gross ignorance and dabbling in matters of life and death as this implies.[70]

But John Packard, a surgeon at the Episcopal Hospital in Philadelphia, was hardly reassured. He strongly supported the idea of formal training schools for nurses, he told an 1876 audience that he hoped might support this agenda. But he had also heard rumors that Nightingale nurses were taught medical anatomy, physiology, pathology, and chemistry and that they learned how to take case histories and dress wounds. Certainly, Packard cautioned, "one could hardly expect the resulting cyclopedia to submit to directions, unless from someone who had a certificate that he knew more than they did."[71] And some formally trained nurses were quite aware that they did, in fact, know more than many practicing physicians who had not the benefit of an elite medical education. As one such nurse wrote of her experiences in Chicago in 1881: "Neither physicians nor people are yet educated up to the idea that the trained nurse is a good thing. The former are fearful we are going, with our diplomas, to open offices and practice medicine, and we think some of us could better do so than many of the so-called doctors who have purchased their diplomas outright, while we have put in the actual two years and more for the knowledge we have gained."[72]

A small but committed cadre of white lay women activists, elite physicians, and women who would be nurses constantly pushed the idea of scientific nursing as subversive to this very kind of doctoring—with its haphazardly organized knowledge, its mediocre training, and its association with the notorious scandals in which, for the proper price, even a child could secure a credential.[73] Moreover, the place for training these nurses would be in hospitals. Nightingale had placed them there when she helped establish the Home and School for Nurses at St. Thomas' in London in 1860. Civil War surgeons had recognized the value of having them there. And those seeking to re-image and reform the institution itself quickly realized they needed them there.

In Philadelphia, Pauline Henry, a scion of New York's prominent van der Kemp family, a philanthropist deeply concerned about women's education and a frequent patient during long bouts of debilitating illnesses, was one such activist. Much as had her female counterparts in Boston, New York, and New Haven, she had long wanted to move such nursing into the most prominent hospitals in the city.[74] But she had less immediate success. She had first offered the University of Pennsylvania $1000 to establish a formal training school in the new hospital it opened in 1872. The Hospital of the University of Pennsylvania (HUP) refused; it preferred a more traditional arrangement in which its house staff assumed responsibility for the observations, the procedures, and the emergencies that occurred during the attending physicians' absences and in which a matron, under the supervision of a philanthropically minded and socially superior Board of Lady Visitors, would be accountable for the nursing and other domestic duties.[75]

Henry had then turned to the Woman's Hospital in 1874 as the only hospital in Philadelphia with a nurses training program in place. But as Henry had written to its Board of Lady Managers during negotiations, she was concerned that its training school experiences were "too limiting" to ensure that nurses were "properly trained." Like other supporters of nursing, Henry envisioned nurses moving beyond an earlier tradition that had certainly celebrated women's medical work but had also confined it to the needs of women and children. Nurses needed the education that placed them within the orbit of all that was new, scientific, and possible. The only limit she placed on her gift was that it had to be used to place Woman's Hospital trained nurses in other Philadelphia hospitals.[76]

The Woman's Hospital accepted Henry's terms and established an experimental affiliation with the Philadelphia Hospital, the city's public hospital. Simultaneously, the Pennsylvania Hospital, the city's oldest and most venerable institution had become more interested in the idea of trained nurses and had tentatively begun its experiment. In 1876 it had hired Fanny Irwin, a Woman's Hospital graduate, as an assistant matron in charge of nursing care. When Irwin resigned in 1877 to return to the Woman's Hospital, Anna Barkely, another graduate, succeeded her in the newly created position of head nurse. In the autumn of 1878,

Anna Bunting and three Woman's Hospital nurses in training assumed responsibility for all the nursing care needed in the Pennsylvania Hospital's Women's Department. Bunting remained as superintendent of nurses and in 1884 graduated the first class of the now formal Pennsylvania Hospital Training School for Nurses.[77]

But by 1886, when the Woman's Hospital Board of Lady Managers paused to celebrate its own contributions to the development of a place for women physicians and nurses, the allure of the Nightingale iconography was newly arrived in the city. The Philadelphia Hospital, struggling to pull itself out of a widely publicized scandal of graft, corruption, and abysmal patient care, made a decision to bring Alice Fisher, a St. Thomas graduate and a woman with an impressive background as the superintendent of nursing of several English hospitals, to Philadelphia to establish a formal training school for nurses at the hospital. It was a controversial decision. Many on the Board of Guardians balked at having to pay her higher salary when a "Philadelphia lady" could be employed for less. But George Childs, the president of the board, felt it was a necessary decision. The hospital needed a concrete symbol of its newfound commitment to its patients. Fisher came only when Childs, enamored with both the myth and the reality of Nightingale reform in England, pledged to pay part of her salary from his own considerable fortune.[78] One year later, HUP chose Charlotte Hugo, another St. Thomas graduate, to establish its training school. The powerfully symbolic image of the "Lady with the Lamp," was deeply enmeshed in mid-nineteenth-century social values, roles, and knowledge. The image was part real, part fantasy, part interpretation, and part need. But it also was one that came late to the painstaking processes surrounding the simultaneous creation of scientific medicine and nursing in nineteenth-century Philadelphia.

In many respects, the late nineteenth century's new ideas about sick nursing simply dressed up old hopes. They still reflected the long-held wish that all nursing women might support the knowledge claims of particular elite or "thinking" physicians because they understood the science upon which it built. Woman's Hospital's physicians, for example, continued to provide lectures on nursing to both their nurses and lay women through the 1890s. And while physicians now spoke in terms of "antisepsis" and "asepsis," or of understanding the course of a fever in terms of the "fastigium," the "defervescence decline," and the "preagnon-istic rise" that signaled the approach of death,[79] their language still wanted to draw women into these physicians' practices and away from that of other kinds of practices and practitioners. Late nineteenth-century physicians, in fact, proffered the same trade of medical knowledge for respected, respectable, and authoritative work in support of their vision of doctoring first proposed earlier in the century.

But women who would nurse for pay had refused that earlier trade. And they remained steadfast in their refusal until the trade carried real meaning—until the trade held the potential to create both respected work and a social identity other than that of domestic servant. Certainly, late nineteenth-century medical knowledge—the anatomical manipulations, the physiological experimentations, the chemical analyses, the microscopic explorations, and the bacteriological advances—had yet to produce the stunning achievements that would ultimately justify faith in a triumphant medicine. But its foundations were in the kinds of learning—in the knowledge of anatomy, physiology, chemistry, and biology—that invited women who would nurse into a world of science now acknowledged as the almost exclusive birthright of the young men and women of middle-class America. And while such women would continue to participate in the late nineteenth century's labor market by exchanging their work for wages, they might differentiate their work from that of working-class white women and all African American women who occupied the bottom rungs of the wage labor hierarchy. White trained nurses could now join white, middle-class men and women in thinking about what they did as work that involved thinking with one's head and not just working with one's hands.[80] As the Farrand Training School explained to its students in 1884, it was work that acknowledged that "merely looking at the sick is not observing. To look is not always to see. It needs a higher degree of training to look, so that looking shall tell the nurse aright."[81] Payments were now made for this specialized intellectual work. Indeed, S. Weir Mitchell assured nurses, accepting payment for one's work did not lessen their status. Rather, payments to them were akin to those to a physician. They only added to the moral as well as to the therapeutic obligations they owed their patients.[82]

Moreover, the hospital as the site of this learning opened up a new public space—one far away from the intimate and private nineteenth-century home. The hospital as classroom would give women who would nurse the ability to differentiate their claims to specialized medical knowledge that were the domain of intellectual male physicians from the claims to sanitary knowledge that were the domain of all women, irrespective, at least theoretically, of race and class. Sanitary knowledge—in empowering all women—only reproduced the established and powerful claims of class, social status, and race of white, middle-class women. By contrast, specialized medical knowledge, taught by powerful physicians and learned in a context dedicated to science and scientific healing, would allow women invited to train as nurses to invest themselves with an authority that might effectively compete with maternal claims at the bedsides of sick patients at home. The real power inherent in the work of trained sick nurses, in fact, lay as much in their new relationship with physicians as in their new relationships with other women—irrespective of these other women's claims of class or social status. Sick nurses would continue to perform the complicated calculus of deciding among competing interests when considering how to care for their patients. But now, as the knowledgeable allies—the authoritative lieutenants—of scientifically minded physicians, their own judgments carried more legitimacy than the opinions of their patients and their families. Sick nurses supported the practices of traditionally trained physicians, and these physicians in turn supported the judgments of nurses working in the homes of mothers who would hire them. Remember, one such physician warned families, once they had made a commitment to a particular nurse—in ways similar to that made to a physician—they must respect it. To question a nurse's knowledge and actions would be to "deny her ability and make her useless."[83]

Certainly not all—and perhaps not most—lay men and women agreed. For some men, the idea of a trained nurse provided a sexualized fantasy.[84] And for some women, the idea of trained nurses provided a wonderful example of one way of addressing the ubiquitous "servant problem." Training schools for domestic servants may seem visionary, one such woman wrote in 1896, but so was once the idea of training schools for nurses. "Brains are required in the kitchen," she continued, as well as in the sick room. "Shall we not have trained servants," she wondered, "when their work demands a like degree of excellence?"[85] Even active supporters of trained nurses felt the need to add some cautionary notes.

"Do not be too particular about your dignity," the lay women and physicians who supported the Nightingale-styled Connecticut Training School for Nurses warned trained nurses in a manual intended both for them and for the mothers who might hire them. "There will be many hours, if your patient is not seriously ill, where, by assisting in the family sewing, or in other ways, you can make yourself useful with things you can bring into the sick room."[86]

This idea of a trained sick nurse reaffirmed the simultaneous racialization and gendering of sick nursing because the image of the trained white female nurse hid from view the continuing place of men and African Americans in the work of caring for the sick. It also stabilized the gender hierarchies threatened by the idea of women as physicians. The idea of a trained female sick nurse, in fact, played particularly well to these gender politics. The "'Woman question' in medicine," Alfred Stille, the president of the AMA, warned in 1871, was akin to "another disease that has become epidemic." It seemed to him "vulgar" that women should be physicians for, he continued, "Is not nursing the chief agent in the cure of disease, and who is so fit a nurse as woman!"[87]

But even as the idea reaffirmed gendered and raced boundaries, it also opened possibilities. The idea of a nurse in a particular kind of relationship with a particular kind of physician represented a more inclusive, in some ways a more open, and certainly a more acceptable articulation of women's relationship with medical knowledge. It embodied a specific form of socially legitimate authority and identity that white women could deploy not only in their relationships with physicians but, just as importantly, in their relationships with other women from their own or other kinds of communities. They were now assistants to men, not mothers. They had the potential power to subvert the practices of some and support the practices of others. In the end, both the idea and the work of a trained sick nurse evolved in the context of negotiated trades in which those who would train as sick nurses would receive as much as they gave.

The idea of a trained sick nurse was in some ways an archetype in writings of Philadelphia's lay and medical men and women. By 1890, there were still fewer than 500 trained nurses across the United States. But it was an idea that ultimately succeeded. By 1900 there were 3,500 trained nurses, and by 1910 there were more than 8,000.[88] The idea elided direct engagement with the cultural ambivalence with which women physicians struggled. It did support explicitly gendered constructions of ideas about who should practice what forms of healing. But for those who would train as sick nurses, the idea represented an opportunity to rethink their identities as well as their work. For them, the idea of trained sick nursing stood as a powerful social and intellectual identity for a life rather than just for a moment in a life.

CHAPTER 2

Competence, Coolness, Courage—and Control

I N 1923, ELIZABETH JONES sought to describe nurses and nursing to the readers of *The Messenger*, a then popular and influential lay magazine. As was typical, Jones began by invoking the spirit of Florence Nightingale, in her mind "the world's greatest nurse." She continued by telling how this spirit inspired the next generation of American nursing leaders to establish training schools, create professional associations, and bring advances in medical science into the lives of families across the nation. The nurse, Jones wrote, was more than a teacher. She both brought advice and embodied it. She was, Jones continued, "looked upon by most of those with whom she comes in contact, as an example of a higher life."[1]

However important the work of nurses, Jones noted, how they did that work was even more significant. She believed a particular combination of content and character defined professional nursing. Content opened the nurse's gaze to the life of an individual "as it really is, and not as it seems to be," and character placed the nurse in a position of trust when dealing with "other problems besides helping to heal the diseased." Certainly, education was important. She told her readers of the "educational unrest" felt by nurses who sought more scientific knowledge about dietetics, pathology, bacteriology, and languages to care for individual patients. But ultimately, she wrote, "it is not the duties we have to perform that count." Nurses and nursing were "impressions," or, as we might say today, representations. It was as much about how one presented oneself as what one did. As an African American nurse, Jones believed that she epitomized the "New Negro Woman." It would be the New Negro Nurse's professional combination of education and disciplined integrity that would force white America, however reluctantly, to acknowledge the African American nurse, and through her all black America's "aptness and talent." Nurses would be among the vanguard, and, she concluded, "eventually [the white man] will be compelled to take us on our merits rather than on our skins."[2]

By the time Jones wrote her article, the ideal of the trained sick nurse had ceded to the reality of formally trained nurses with credentials from training schools in hospitals throughout the country. The experiment with such training schools had begun slowly. In 1880, fifteen hospitals had established training schools; by 1890, only twenty more had followed suit. By 1900, however, the numbers had grown to 432 such schools as real advances in aseptic techniques turned hospitals into preferred sites for surgery and, increasingly, for childbirth. The numbers of training schools then tripled, to 1,129 by 1910 before stabilizing at approximately 1,700 to 1,800 through the 1920s.[3] There were training schools in large urban hospitals as well as in small rural ones. Women's hospitals, children's hospitals, and tuberculosis sanatoriums had training schools. Most such schools admitted only single white women, although a small number also admitted one or two women of color. Most African American women who would be nurses trained in the small but growing numbers of training schools established by African American hospitals. Men who would nurse trained in insane asylums.

In the opening decades of the twentieth century, there were as yet few standards for what a training school should teach and how it should be structured. Each individual training school was, in the words of one nursing educator, a "law unto itself." It was established by, responsible to, and reflective of the priorities and preferences of a particular hospital's board of directors.[4] But they all had the same form. Student nurses, under the direction of a nursing superintendent, provided all the hospital's nursing work. Much like hospital medical students and house staff, they bartered their time and their nursing work for the knowledge, the clinical opportunities, and the credentials they received in exchange.[5] Upon graduation, they left the hospital for work in homes and health care agencies across the country. Upcoming and incoming students took their place.

This training school experience emphasized medical science, skilled techniques, discipline, loyalty, obedience, and the acceptance, even the embrace, of a gendered place within a hierarchical medical structure. At its worst, the training school experience easily deteriorated into negligible time in lecture halls, absurdly strict discipline, blind loyalty, and rote obedience. But at its best, the experience provided the knowledge, training, and support that relatively young and inexperienced women needed when confronted—many, for the first time in their lives—with the responsibility for managing the often overwhelming encounters with their patients' pain, suffering, sexuality, and death. It offered the social and psychological context within which admittedly unpleasant body work—changing bloodied dressings, catheterizing male patients, cleaning vomit, urine, and feces—might be reframed. This work would now become, in the words of one nursing educator, an almost religious "sacrifice" of both one's own feelings of propriety and, in that this work sometimes meant inflicting pain, one's patient's feeling of comfort.[6] Elizabeth Jones's impressions were honed by three years of such an education.

Certainly, African American women like Jones, and white women who were the vast majority of students, came to nurses' training with widely different backgrounds and experiences. But this chapter explores what they shared by the time they graduated from their respective schools. It turns to a small group of early twentieth-century white, middle-class nursing educators who appropriated control of particular elements of the training school experience and ultimately fashioned a new and different relationship between themselves, medical knowledge, and clinical practice. This relationship certainly embodied the traits of discipline, loyalty, and obedience. But, this chapter argues, such traits served in the production of more important representations, or, in Jones' words, "impressions": those of competence, coolness, courage, and control of clinical spaces. Such representations came from a self-consciously constructed approach to both medical content and individual character.[7] They also provided the foundation for trained nurses' claims of expertise. And, this chapter continues, such representations created an internalized and fairly stable conceptualization of a strong nursing identity, albeit one shaded by the multiple meanings of a nurse's particular world.

Educating Women

Trained nursing may have been born in the trade of knowledge for work between physicians and women who would nurse, but it came of age as increasing numbers of women sought and received more formal education, including collegiate education. As Barbara Miller Solomon has argued, the period between the 1870s and the opening decades of the twentieth century witnessed an "extraordinary movement of women" into institutions of higher education either designed specifically for them or finally opening their doors to them. In 1870, 59 percent of all colleges accepted only men, and only 29 percent were coeducational. By 1910, the percentage of colleges only admitting men had plummeted to 27 percent, while the percentage of coeducational institutions had soared to 58 percent. Granted, the numbers of women enrolled remained small: only 0.7 percent of all women between the ages of eighteen and twenty-one were enrolled in college in 1870 and only 3.8 percent by 1910.[8] In fact, collegiate education was a part of only 5 percent of all Americans' experiences.[9] But both the awareness and the fact of women's presence on collegiate campuses was unmistakable. While they accounted for only 21 percent of all enrollments in 1870, they represented almost 40 percent of all students by 1910.[10]

These numbers played themselves out within a complicated matrix of race, religion, ethnicity, geography, and culture that invited some women in, left some women out, and created a certain ambivalence—if no longer overt hostility—in other women's lives. The experience of private and philanthropically supported colleges such as Radcliffe, Vassar, and Bryn Mawr remained one available almost exclusively to white, Protestant women of a certain privileged social background. Many African American women, women with foreign-born parents, Jewish and Catholic women, women remaining near their southern-born roots, and women from families without privileged backgrounds found their way to any higher education institution with difficulty.[11]

Part of the issue, of course, was the enmeshment of women's quest for additional education in what Solomon has called a fundamental "historical paradox"—women taking increased advantage of new opportunities not always designed for them in a context that still privileged the education of men over that of women.[12] Among both Catholics and white southerners, for example, one saw families taking the progressive position of supporting their daughters' educational ambitions—while sending them to single-sex sectarian institutions because of their concern that coeducation might be detrimental to the education of their sons.[13] Among the

African American and Irish Catholic middle class, in particular—where a collegiate experience was an increasingly accepted, if not expected, part of the social experience of many of their daughters—the emphasis remained on education in the service of privileging women's traditional roles as educated ladies, mothers, and, if one needed to support one's self or one's family, as teachers, librarians, and social workers.[14]

Still, questions continued about who might have access to college education and, perhaps more importantly, for what purposes. Edward Clarke, a retired professor from Harvard's medical school, first raised these questions in what would become the infamous *Sex in Education,* published in 1873. Women, he argued, may have an individual right to higher education, but this right posed significant risks to their biological role in childbearing. When inherently limited physiological energy was used in studying, he concluded in a study based on seven Vassar graduates, it compromised their reproductive capabilities. But while it was widely read and discussed, the flurry of excitement generated by this book subsided quickly. Its conclusions were alternately ridiculed and convincingly refuted by women physicians and social scientists. And any worries it created were quickly replaced by those suggesting that middle-class women's academic grades, awards, and accomplishments might soon outstrip those of their male classmates.[15]

Ambivalence about the implications of enlightening and broadening liberal education in the lives of American women persisted. Collegiate education had a firm place in some women's lives, but it continued to create anxiety about its destabilizing possibilities. S. Weir Mitchell perfectly captured such concerns in his address to the students of Radcliffe College, Harvard's sister institution, in 1895. He charmed and flattered his audience, speaking as both a physician and a fellow man of science and letters. He told them clearly that higher education was never, in and of itself, a cause of physical or emotional suffering: "I believe that most women would be wiser, better, and therefore happier, for larger intellectual training." But if women had the same freedom and rights as did their brothers, they now had the same responsibilities in the exercise of such privileges. In the end, both men and women had to assume responsibility for exercising their privileges "within the noble limitations" of their gender. "I personally no more want them [women] to be preachers, lawyers, or platform orators, then I want men to be seamstresses or nurses of children," he added.[16]

Mitchell looked much more approvingly upon nurses' education. "In the evolution of American women," he proclaimed in a 1908 commencement address to the graduates of the Hospital of the University of Pennsylvania Training School for Nurses, "your training is the one advance in education about which there can be no doubt concerning what it gives, and no sad conviction as to what it misses or takes away." Mitchell waxed eloquently to the graduates: "Yours is the only profession which ideally benefits the woman; yours is the only education which takes all that is best, morally and naturally, and educates it so as to prepare you for the woman's life, the nurse business, the wife business, motherhood."[17] One can hear Mitchell's pomposity and condescension—artifacts of his class, patriarchal, and professional place. One can celebrate the accomplishments of other women who successfully challenged his circumscribed ideas about women's proper place and roles. But one must still take seriously the salience of his ideas about the social implications of nursing education: about its resonance with particularly strong and enduring ideas about women's roles in their families and communities.

Training Nurses

Mitchell might also have added that nursing education was perhaps the most predominant of all new higher educational opportunities available to a much broader range of American women, one specifically designed for them and accessible to them, and one that privileged their education over that of their brothers. Certainly, American nursing leaders claimed such for their training schools. Isabel Hampton Robb, one of the most powerful and persuasive of fin de siècle American nursing leaders, proclaimed nurses unique in that they were the first women to be provided with the complete training of the hands, the head, and the heart that were the core of all women's educational aspirations.[18]

Robb, a Canadian-born music teacher, had fled her home for New York City and the excitement and the opportunity that awaited newly trained nurses. She had graduated from the city's prestigious Bellevue Hospital Training School in 1883, and, when not nursing sick English and American travelers at a small hospital in Rome, had traveled through Europe. She returned to the United States to assume the position as head of the Illinois Training School for Nurses at Chicago's Cook County Hospital in 1886.[19] Three years later, she arrived in Baltimore as the first superintendent of the new Johns Hopkins Hospital Training School for Nurses. This hospital, Robb's biographer Janet James reminds us, drew from German experiences and was deliberately created as a model American hospital in which patient care would be closely related to medical teaching and research. It was one in which nurses would be part of a community of science within the hospital. At the ceremony inaugurating the training school in October 1889, Henry Hurd, the medical superintendent of the hospital, promised that in its coursework, in its clinical training, and in the eyes of the trustees, "nursing the sick is not to be considered a trade but a learned profession."[20]

In Robb's vision, it would be a learned profession *for women*. In her address to physicians, philanthropists, and other professionals committed to improvements in health and social welfare at the general session of the International Congress of Charities, Correction, and Philanthropy at the Chicago World's Fair of 1893, she spoke of the meaning of nursing to women and of their roles, their work, and their responsibilities. "Can a women, in any other kind of work which she may chose for herself," she wondered, "find a higher ideal or a graver responsibility" than that of nursing—than that of dedicating one's life to the preservation of human life and the alleviation of human suffering. Trained nurses, she explained, cared for the sick in the homes of both private families and the urban poor. Just as importantly, nurses who so wished also had new opportunities for entrée to religious missions abroad and medical schools at home. But however they served, their commitment was to participate in the "progress that is medical science"—albeit with their particular part to perform. Nurses were, she graciously conceded, "only the handmaid of that great and beautiful science in whose temple she may only serve in minor parts." She shared with her audience a metaphor in a physician's address to a graduating class of trained nurses. "The hands of the nurses," she approvingly quoted, "are the physician's hands lengthened out to minister to the sick. Her watchful vigilance at the bedside is a trained vigilance supplementing and perfecting his watchful care; her knowledge of his patient's condition an essential element in the diagnosis of disease; her management of the patient, the practical side of medical science."[21]

Robb willingly cast nursing as a hierarchical handmaiden—but not necessarily to physicians. Science mediated gendered relationships. Nurses' roles were played in relation to a form of science that as easily claimed men in similarly hierarchical relationships within the temple as its worshipful priests. It accepted graciously set, properly deferential, and publicly acknowledged performances at the bedsides of sick patients—but claimed its own physical and emotional work with patients as a medium to both engage with science and to act as scientists.[22] Nursing, in Robb's words, had an absolute "duty" to science, and each nurse must "grasp the import of its teachings, that she may fulfill wisely her share."[23]

The Relationship between Nursing and Science

Science content was certainly necessary to the knowledge claims made by nurses like Elizabeth Jones.[24] Physicians taught nurses anatomy, physiology, bacteriology, psychology, neurology, and social hygiene. Martha Collett Soper's 1919 and 1920 lecture notes give some sense of the content taught nurses at leading American training schools like her alma mater, the Hospital of the University of Pennsylvania Training School for Nurses. During her first year in training, Soper learned about normal and abnormal cell metabolism, bone structure, and muscle physiology. She studied the vascular system, the lymphatic system, the respiratory system, and the nervous system. Soper also attended lectures about digestive system metabolism and about the attendant correlations between particular anabolic and catabolic processes and the proper selection of therapeutic foods and drinks. Like most nursing students, Soper attended lectures in addition to her responsibilities to the hospital's patients, and her lecture notes were reviewed for accuracy by her nursing instructor. She may well have been exhausted from both her ward work and her class work on the day that the circulatory system was presented. "Circulation takes place by the veins," she wrote in her notes. "No," her instructor wrote back, "return circulation takes place there."[25]

If necessary, such science content was not sufficient. Nurses' command of the facts of certain areas of science was often matched, if not often exceeded, by that of other educated men and women. As one Dr. Hamilton P. Jones reminded students at New Orleans Charity Hospital's Training School for Nurses in 1912, the aggressive publicizing of new scientific discoveries by both medical and lay presses had already given families in general, and patients in particular, up-to-date knowledge about the "germ diseases" and the use of serums, vaccines, isolation, quarantine, nursing, and dietetics in their treatment. Thus nurses, he warned, needed to always make sure they were "armed" with "proper and accurate knowledge" when they practiced in such homes.[26]

Annie Goodrich, one of the leading nursing voices in the campaign to provide some standardization of the widely varying training school experience, painted a starker picture. Goodrich had been a staunchly reform-minded superintendent of several prominent New York City training schools. She now lectured at Teachers College, Columbia University, and had just been appointed the New York state inspector of training schools. She was working tirelessly to establish mandatory standards in nurses' training schools, and she wanted and needed a broader base of support for her campaign.[27] "It is humiliating to state," she told an audience of hospital administrators, "and yet I believe it to be a fact, that many graduates of domestic science know more about nutrition than those professionally prepared to deal with health or disease."[28] She also appealed to her physician colleagues. Some schools, she told members of the New York Academy of Medicine, did produce nurses with authority and expert knowledge. But many more, if not most schools, produced nurses at a distinct disadvantage. They produced nurses, she argued, with less knowledge about hygiene and sanitation than, as she put it, "lay students in high school or those reading popular magazines."[29]

Goodrich, like most American nursing leaders, desperately wanted to see their potential student nurses as, at the least, like the white, middle-class high school girl who had the extra money to spend on popular magazines. They wanted such students to be ambitious, socially conscious, and reform-minded women like themselves. Goodrich's intimate social circle included both nurses Adelaide Nutting, the director of the first postgraduate nursing program at Columbia's Teachers College, and Lillian Wald, the founder of the Henry Street Settlement House. By day, the nurses who lived and worked at Henry Street attended to the health and illness needs of the working poor and immigrants living around them in New York City's lower east side. By night, they strategized new reforms with the lay and medical friends who lived with them for longer or shorter periods of time. Such friends included S. Josephine Baker, the first female medical examiner for the New York City Health Department, who was deeply concerned with the health of the poorest of the city's children. In fact, as Baker recalled in her memoir, *Fighting for Life*, Goodrich, Wald, and she belonged to so many of the same reform committees that a reporter, finding them again together on yet another evening, wanted only to know, "What are you calling yourselves tonight?"[30]

This same social consciousness informed Goodrich's assessment of the current state of nursing in general, and nursing education in particular. Certainly, she, like many other of her nursing colleagues, could be harsh about the fact that most incoming students seemed to fall short of their white, middle-class ideal. Hospitals had quickly realized the economic and clinical value of students willing to trade their work for knowledge, and they set entrance requirements at levels that would attract the numbers of students needed to staff its wards. These requirements varied widely as each hospital carefully balanced the numbers of students needed with the minimum educational background needed to learn to nurse. In many, if not most cases, these requirements were well below what nursing leadership felt was necessary. Should a young girl, Goodrich wondered before an audience of students at New York City's Metropolitan Training School in 1912, moreover, a girl with only an elementary school education, as was sometimes the case, be the "sole guardian of ten or twenty acutely sick patients at night?"[31] Like most American nursing leaders, she laid much blame at the feet of hospitals for their tight control over, and narrow vision of, their respective training schools. But Goodrich also turned her sights on what seemed to her to be the alarming lack of concern, if not the utter indifference, of the community to the fact that the training schools failed to attract well-educated students. How is it, she wondered, that the community "does . . . not yet grasp the increasing dissatisfaction of young women with our training schools for nurses?"[32]

Nursing's leadership also wished and actively campaigned for an educational system that de-emphasized the power of the hospital and its almost insatiable demands for patient care, that allowed more concentrated time for didactic instruction, and that increasingly replicated that of collegiate education taking hold for women. Still, they constantly recognized one essential difference between their mission in their training schools and that of other educators in colleges. "We do not stand in the position of colleges and universities," Nutting wrote in 1898. A degree or diploma from such institutions, she continued, promised only that its holder knew certain facts, demonstrated certain competencies, and had achieved a certain degree of education. It did not attest to the holder's temperament, personality, or disposition. "We stand in a different and peculiar situation," she noted. The nursing diploma testified to certain facts, competencies, and education. But it also bore witness to its holder's character: she would put patients' needs before her own, faithfully execute medical orders, hold sick-bed confidences in trust, and provide calming experiences that would put suffering minds at ease. "We assume," she concluded, "a moral responsibility for the character of the nurses we send out."[33]

Moreover, nursing's leadership argued, the public expected nurses to assume such responsibilities. By the early twentieth century, criticisms of the trained nurse were rampant as an idea gave way to reality. Physicians who needed trained nurses for their patients, for example, complained about their slowness in responding to calls. Families who employed them complained about their fees. And even the nursing educators who trained them complained about their blithe interruption of household routines while nursing private patients.[34]

But in all honesty, these same educators pointed out, how much of this critique might be attributable to nurses per se, and how much might be a reflection of the public's general uneasiness with the idea of the "new woman," who increasingly turned her back on traditional domestic skills, preferring to experiment with more exciting ones needed in a workforce increasingly open to them? The "glaring imperfections" laid at the feet of nurses, Robb noted, were amply shared with other working women. Nurses, she continued, might indeed suffer from the plague of "inefficiency and a lack of thoroughness." But such traits belonged, not to the graduate nurse alone, but they were "the common property of the modern woman."[35] Where the public might tolerate the shortcomings of other "professional" women, however, it would not tolerate them in nurses. Nurses, most if not all leaders and educators believed, were and should be held to a "higher standard" of morality. They, and they alone, were privileged with duties of a much higher importance and ones that involved both "the great problems of life and the mysteries of death and suffering."[36]

The Relationship between Content and Character

The "higher standard," of course, included every known, feminized, and idealized Victorian character trait. The woman who would be a nurse had to be, first, virtuous, honest, faithful, truthful, sympathetic, tactful, gentle, sweet, devout, loyal, obedient, and, ultimately, worthy of the place she sought in a middle-class American household. She would be a "lady of culture" as well as a skilled professional, creating, through her nature, an "alchemy of influence" critical to her patient's healing and health.[37] This discourse preoccupied the nursing superintendents of training schools most directly responsible for producing this putative saint. They endlessly debated among themselves whether such traits were inherent or learned, and they bemoaned—sometimes touchingly, sometimes annoyingly—the lack of the "right kind of women" in the profession.

In many respects they did so because as educators they had little direct control over the medical content taught their students. This was taught by physicians and depended upon an individual physician's time, interest, and availability. Furthermore, medical content was itself embedded within an even more complicated social matrix that included both the race of the practitioner and the local—and relative—place of practice. African American nurses, for example, most often trained in resource-starved African American hospitals where they had fewer options to expand upon the content of their scientific education and fewer opportunities to experience latest scientific tools and techniques. In addition, most southern trained nurses—African American or white— found themselves at a disadvantage vis-à-vis northern trained nurses. Northern cities had larger and more established hospitals as well as a more developed public and private educational infrastructure that placed all northern trained professional women—teachers and social workers as well as nurses—at a distinct advantage.[38] Moreover, the medical content available to nurses who trained in the smaller hospitals that concentrated on surgical and obstetrical cases most often focused only on the particular needs of the patients under care, ignoring much broader content that would be needed in their practices after graduation. The same was true for nurses who trained in specialized hospitals such as children's hospitals, tuberculosis sanitariums, or insane asylums. Sometimes it seemed as if the education depended solely on the initiative of the individual student. "I don't know what is the matter with this patient," Dorothy Green wrote in her probationer's diary in 1899, "but I am trying to be very observing and find things out for myself. . . . I noticed Miss Junior poured a lot of medicine in her hair . . . and I noticed that the label read 'Delphinium,' so I must look it up and see what it is used for."[39]

But nursing educators did control their students' day-to-day experiences, and they paid close attention to the formative processes that would turn a feminized ideal—or as close an approximation as they could attract to their school—into a trained nurse. These experiences involved the application of medical content learned in lectures and the careful development of skilled nursing techniques. It also involved learning, applying, and appropriating the new language of scientific medicine. It meant, as Martha Collett Soper recorded in her lecture notes, to consider pneumonia not just as a "germ disease" but as one that needed a more careful, more precise, and more expressive vocabulary that included such terms as pneumococcal bacteria, toxemia, blood profusion, hepatization, pleura, aspiration, and empyrema.[40] It meant, as nursing's *materia medica* textbooks pointed out, that medication administration needed to be calculated in terms of grains and drachms, not drops or spoonfuls.[41] And it meant, when describing the results of vigilant observations, to remember that listening to the body would now be termed "auscultation," that a noted difficulty in breathing would be called "dyspnea," and the sounds of digestion needed to be described as "peristalsis."[42]

In many ways, learning this new language was the crux of nurses' education in medical content. As anthropologist Bryon Good has argued, learning the language of medicine consisted, not of learning new words for the commonsense world, but in learning to use these new words to construct an entirely new world of meaning and experience.[43] The quality of education in medical content could indeed vary. But learning the language of medical content enabled women to enter the domain of science, objectivity, rationality, and reasoned action. As historian Joan Lynaugh has suggested, learning this new language allowed nurses to "know" what they saw and to then act upon what they knew with knowledge and authority.[44] And it allowed nurses to know and to act in a more depersonalized and detached manner.

Discipline and Detachment

Discipline was the cornerstone of the day-to-day formative experiences that brought a woman into this new world of meaning and transformed her into a trained nurse. The weeks and months of disciplined drilling and repetitions were self-consciously in the service of creating the "automatic" responses that allowed for no hesitation in the face of crises, no discrimination when confronted with patients whose behavior one abhorred, and no questioning in the face of a superior's orders.[45] Granted, such drillings and repetitions, as acts in and of themselves, could be and often were carried too far. As one educator pointed out, one could only learn such things as expert bed-making (something of real comfort to a critically ill patient) through constant repetitions, but she also wondered if it was necessary to make thousands of beds to learn this one skill.[46]

Some students found the focus on disciplined procedures a bulwark against a loss of individuality and a "hardening" of the self to a patient's pain and suffering. Nell Peckens Pease struggled with this throughout her training at Bellevue. She wrote long, thoughtful, and reflective letters to her fiancé in Pennsylvania, worrying that her distaste for the poor, pregnant, and unmarried women on the obstetric wards of the hospital would overwhelm her sense of herself as kind, gentle, and compassionate. Some of her patients, she admitted, were "very refined and ashamed." But most were "rough and coarse, and have not the slightest bit of shame and modesty." Sometimes, she admitted, "I almost despise myself and all mankind . . . and have been afraid that the place will get the best of me—and yet I have worked hard not to let it." The discipline and the regularity of her training helped her cope. Still, she continued, "I sometimes wonder if you will find me changed much when I get home."[47]

These weeks and months of disciplined drilling and repetitions were self-consciously militaristic. But the militaristic analogies were also re-appropriated. They were now not merely Samuel Gross's "lieu-tenants." They were now akin to West Point and Annapolis cadets—officers in training preparing for future leadership roles.[48] The militaris-tic protocols were likewise fairly well delineated within nursing in terms of experience and expertise. The probationer stood in the presence of the junior student, who stood in the presence of and deferred to the senior student, who, in turn, stood in the presence of and deferred to the head nurse—who may or may not have been a student. The head nurse was responsible for everything that occurred on her ward, and it was the duty of all other less-skilled and less-experienced students to keep her informed. But it was also the responsibility of these students to rise to the head nurses' expectations. Disciplined drillings and repetitions helped students build the skill and confidence to do so. Dorothy Green recalled that after her head nurse had reviewed the night orders with her, the one and only thought in her mind was *How am I going to accomplish it all?* But, she remembered, there was little time for asking unanswerable questions. She knew how to handle the reality that she had "a dozen PRN orders [for medications that depended on the nurse's judgment] to be attended to at once; half-hourly hypodermic injections to one patient, hourly poultices to another, hot compresses to another; and three patients on this ward had little babies, to whom nourishment was given every three to four hours." She also knew she had "three para-lytic patients needing almost constant care, and one old lady who was in the habit of taking midnight strolls and had to have a sharp eye kept upon her, for all the patients feared the ghost-like form of old Bridget in her little short gown and huge carpet slippers."[49]

In keeping with protocol, all nurses stood "like a sentinel on duty" in the presence of physicians. This, Robb noted, needed to be tempered with "common sense." Nurses could hardly keep rising every time any one of a number of physicians constantly moving in and out of the wards all day decided to look in on his patient.[50] In addition, these protocols—in ways we have not yet completely recognized—involved an entire sys-tem of deference, control, accommodation, and communication that involved more than just nurse/nurse and physician/nurse dyads.

Physicians, for example, had established their own protocols when involved with consulting physicians. Their 1912 code of ethics—as much a statement of ethical principles as a code of professional conduct—

advocated "tactfulness" in the relationship and carefully warned against the "insincerity, rivalry, or envy" that might invade it. In ways that echoed of nurses' ethical prohibitions against challenging medical diagnoses and treatments, the medical code prohibited consultants from directly sharing their opinions with patients.[51] In cases of unsolvable or nonnegotiable disagreements that the code's elaborate arbitration procedures failed to resolve, the consulting physician had to do precisely what *Nursing Ethics* set forth for nurses in similar disagreements with physicians: first withdraw from the case, and then set forth one's opinion to the patient or family paying one's fee.[52] In many respects, patients were the lowest players on the proverbial stage. As one nurse wrote of her training school experience: a nurse never need submit to the rudeness or insults of patients; if he or she persisted in such behavior, she reported, the patient would be discharged. But, she did add, "a very sick patient is seldom beyond endurance."[53]

Competence and Coolness

But the militaristic processes surrounding discipline were even more important in the articulation and the integration of a detached persona during the clinical moment when a patient needed a nurse's care. First, a nurse learned never to allow any of her feelings about her patient or her patient's condition to interfere with her own observations, judgment, or treatment. "We have no dreaming time," one told a journalist in 1890, "and there is very little place for sentiment, and very little sympathy in the ordinary sense of the word." She did not want to appear too harsh to the lay audience that would read her words. "Were we to sympathize with all the woes that we see," she explained, "we should be used up and we should die."[54]

In sharp contrast to the qualities of the putative saint that pervaded the popular literature, an effective nurse had to learn to be, as one 1899 textbook explained, "strong-nerved and of steady hand." More pragmatically, she had to be "habituated to the sight of blood," but above all, self-possessed and never obviously surprised, caught unaware, or thrown off her guard.[55] She may have appropriated maternal images, but she was not the patient's mother. Indeed, Lavinia Dock, an avowed feminist, determined suffragette, and one of the most outspoken and progressive of nursing's early leaders, spoke for many nurses when she sometimes regarded mothers as allies in the care of particular patients but most often believed them to be her opponents. Mothers, she wrote in 1903, were too often "nerveless and weak-hearted" when they needed to give their child an uncomfortable treatment. They were "doubly ineffective," she pronounced, "when the orders call for treatment so distinctly repugnant as nasal irrigation, throat spraying, and the like." The nurse simply held the child firmly, steadily, and insistently. The mother, by contrast, threw up her arms and delivered the "stereotyped" answer: "He won't let me."[56]

But knowledge for competent clinical care also involved more than just the ability to understand, explain, and execute prescribed treatments proficiently and calmly. Indeed, as one physician lecturer correctly noted, many of the nurses' more "ordinary duties"—taking temperatures, administering medications, bathing patients, preparing therapeutic diets, or preparing a sick room—might be accomplished by almost any "intelligent" person motivated to learn the basics of home nursing care.[57] Nurses' knowledge involved much more. It involved wanting to learn such basics and taking pride in the skilled techniques with which they delivered them. More importantly, however, nurses' knowledge allowed them to understand the *implications* of the resulting data, and their coolness in assessing such implications enabled them to form judgments about how to proceed—in ways which may or may not have conformed to prescribed treatments. Nurses would follow orders— but not mindlessly or rigidly. Nurses would be watchful and waiting— but when necessary, they would also act immediately, forcefully, and competently.

The cool, detached, competent, and disciplined clinical performances in the face of rapid clinical deterioration or medical emergencies were, of course, the most dramatic moments on which nurses built their knowledge claims. These knowledge claims did present something of a quandary. They were built on moments that were often invisible to patients and their families. Indeed, the better the nursing care, the less likely such moments would occur. They were also built upon moments that happened only infrequently and hence were much less noticeable to outsiders than the day-to-day processes involving more routine nursing care. But within the tightly bounded world of physicians and nurses, there was never any doubt of the validity of such claims. Success or failure in such moments, they both agreed, depended solely upon the independent decisions and the skillful responses of nurses. As educator Agnes Brennan noted, a woman without formal nurses training may become a good nurse, but she could never become an intelligent one. Should an emergency arise, she wondered, "where is she? She is lost: she only knows how to work through her feelings, not through her carefully honed judgment."[58]

When caring for a patient with a "heart disease," for example, a nurse learned that a weakening or "smaller" pulse signaled an imminent crisis that could not wait for the physician's attendance. She had to immediately administer a "stimulating" drug—perhaps camphor, digitalis, or nitroglycerine—to save her patient's life. Or if caring for a patient with pneumonia, she learned that a "crisis," or, in lay terms, a sudden drop in her patient's temperature, needed all her knowledge and judgment. Nurse Maud Banfield wrote from a determination to render the knowledge and skill of trained nurses more visible to the readers of the *Ladies Home Journal*. When a fever crisis struck, the nurse had to immediately replace ice packs with blankets and hot water bottles; change the soaked linens and clothes; maintain absolute quiet, and constantly watch for the signs of collapse and heart failure—of cold noses and ears and an almost imperceptible pulse—that called for the immediate administration of drugs such as whiskey, ammonia, strychnia.[59] Equally dreaded were new mothers' postpartum hemorrhages. Before the physician arrived, the nurse would have changed the patient's position by raising her feet and lowering her head, applied abdominal massage to force uterine contractions, packed the vagina with gauze to staunch bleeding, and administered a hypodermic of ergot.[60] The constant rhetoric, in the words of one lecturer, was that the nurse "should never assume responsibility beyond her sphere."[61] But watchful waiting was no longer good enough. A nurse had to act in the face of sudden changes in her patient's condition, and to act immediately with knowledge, with control, and with authority.

Courage and Control of the Clinical Moment

Still, militaristic processes went beyond just disciplined performance in the clinical moment. Such processes were life-saving. But where some looked toward the safety of the patient, others looked to that of the nurse. Late nineteenth-century women who would be nurses certainly required a certain moral courage in the still socially problematic care of male strangers. But their early twentieth-century successors also needed the physical courage to, in their words, confront, do battle with, and eventually win the war against infectious diseases—diseases that threatened their patients' lives and their own well-being. The new knowledge about infectious diseases and how they were transmitted fundamentally transformed the relationship between nurses and their patients. Patients were no longer the objects of disease or of an infectious bacteria's particular virulence. Rather, they were the *source* of the disease—and the source of a virulent infectious process that could and did encroach upon the well-being of innocent bystanders only trying to help. Nurses, in fact, knew that the strangers they pledged to help could also kill them. Some nurses knew of other nurses who had died; all knew of those who had become ill.[62]

As historian Jeanne Kisacky has argued, early twentieth-century hospitals (and certainly most of the larger, older, and more urban ones) had moved away from Nightingalian notions of light, air, and cleanliness as tools in the battle against the spread of infectious diseases. These institutions, building upon the new bacteriological and epidemiological sciences, now emphasized the importance of physical barriers and elaborate procedural rules to prevent the physical transfer of germs from patients to other people.[63] D. L. Richardson, then the medical superintendent of Providence City Hospital in Rhode Island, recapitulated both the science and the practice in his 1915 article in the *American Journal of Nursing*. Research, he argued, had shown that the notion of "air infection" had been "greatly overrated." Laboratory results certainly demonstrated the presence of some "disease germs" in the air and dust and on the floors and walls of hospitals and sick rooms. But both science and, just as importantly, "practical experience" showed such to be of "small significance" when compared with the problem of the infectious contact—either directly through the bodily secretions and excretions, or indirectly through hands, utensils, or linens that moved from one patient to another.[64] Minnie Goodnow, another leading educator, was more succinct. Nurses, she reminded her colleagues in 1916, had to "stop being afraid of the air." Instead, she argued, we have to "become more careful about our hands."[65]

The 1924 *Nursing Procedure Book* of the Philadelphia General Hospital (PGH) carefully laid out how nurses would act to protect themselves. PGH, as did many institutions, used both physical and procedural barriers to contain infectious contacts. Screens marked the boundary between clean and infectious areas, and carefully delineated procedures described the proper ways of attending to patients within such infectious areas. To assess the vital signs—the temperature, pulse, and respirations—of a patient with cerebro-spinal meningitis, for example, the nurse had to remove her watch and place it on a table outside the infected area. She then had to reach inside the infectious area to get a specially designated gown, being careful to touch only the clean inside (rather than the potentially contaminated outside) of the gown. After "gowning" (a procedure with its own technique to ensure that the gown's contaminated outside never touched the nurse's own uniform), but still outside the infectious area, the nurse had to disinfect her hands in a 2 percent Lysol solution. Next, less there be any confusion, she would take the thermometer in her right hand and her watch in her left and then enter the infectious area. She would place the thermometer in the patient's mouth with her right hand, and, with the same hand, count the pulse with the watch in the "uncontaminated" left hand (to keep it free from inadvertent contact with any infectious materials). This procedure would be repeated six to ten times each day for each infectious patient in her care.

PGH's procedure took some unexpected events into account. "In any instance," the policy continued, "where the nurse must use both hands"—for example, to help the patient sit up in bed—"the pulse should be taken first, the watch replaced on the table outside the area before an attempt is made to take the temperature."[66] But there were no established procedures for most unanticipated incidents: for a patient's coughing spasm as she removed the thermometer, for a nurse's stumble with an armful of soiled linen, or for an unexpected emergency that needed an immediate response. Tuberculosis was a debilitating and sometimes deadly occupational hazard.[67] But nurses, and particularly nurses in training, also struggled against contracting diphtheria infections, scarlet fever, and measles.

In fact, as Goodrich pointed out, while everyone might agree on what should be done, the reality remained that many, if not most, hospitals did not have the physical capacity to do what needed to be done. Too many still had inadequate facilities for disinfecting or destroying infectious materials, and too many had designated "infectious wards" still directly connected to dining rooms and diet kitchens.[68] "Barriered patients" needed to rest within "barrier systems." But systems might be as elaborate as special screens surrounding beds or as simple as tags or tapes on beds alerting staff to maintain aseptic techniques.[69] They might also be jury-rigged systems. Sister Frieda, a deaconess nurse, described the combination bassinet and dressing cabinet she and her colleagues devised to provide individualized isolation care without having the room to create specialized isolation spaces for the infants in their charge. Each little patient now slept in a self-contained and movable bassinet. In the event of an infection—impetigo was especially problematic—the entire cabinet in which each patient lay could be moved away from other infants to another part of the hospital.[70] The theory was known, but the devil was in the implementation details. As one physician noted, there seemed little use in isolating a diphtheria patient if her family were allowed to come and go at will without obtaining any data about their infectious states.[71]

But if cool, detached, and disciplined clinical performance enabled nurses to learn how to independently and assertively control clinical moments, such performances, in the face of infectious diseases, now allowed them to learn to control the clinical spaces in which such moments occurred. They learned to monitor such spaces with tightly regulated visiting hours. They practiced scanning such spaces with a carefully trained eye to make sure everything and everybody was in their proper place. These women learned how to tame the chaos of sickrooms and wards—places of stagnant air, foul smells, contaminated effusions, pitiful sufferings, and searing pain—by following routines, systematizing procedures, and honing disciplined command hierarchies with rules both for following orders and for taking charge. Medical content and medical language fused to reframe the work of these women. "How hopeless and dull, not to say irritating," Robb admitted, "would be the many washings and various aseptic precautions which are now required from the nurse . . . unless she had learned from bacteriology to appreciate the fact that there exists a surgical, microscopic cleanliness."[72] Indeed, the constant emphasis on the orderliness of the well-made bed, well-executed procedure, and well-run ward involved more than the installation of mindless and rote behavior. It also reflected the nurse's need to learn how to rescue patients in environments that sometimes seemed to veer out of their control. The entire sickness experience was always fraught with anxiety and apprehension. As one physician noted, perhaps only those who had experienced the hopelessness and chaos of an illness could appreciate the exactness and the precision that came with the formal training of women as nurses.[73]

Nurses' detached and proficient performances in clinical moments and clinical spaces had social as well as clinical importance. These particular performances may have been learned at the hospital bedside when they were students, but they were enacted by graduate nurses in the homes of both rich families (as private duty nurses) and poor families (as visiting or public health nurses) across the country. Moreover, they were performed at crowded bedsides that included not only physicians, patients, and nurses but also mothers, families, and friends. And they were set on a stage that still had a place for the traditions of a domestic medical culture. This culture, in the eyes of both physicians and trained nurses, still placed too much emphasis on the value of easily obtained medications recommended by friends, on relatively approximate measures of precisely prescribed medications, and on cavalier notions about how and when such medications and treatments might be administered. As the 1926 graduates of the nursing school at the Children and Women's Hospital in San Francisco wrote in their yearbook, they were moving from the hospital into a wider world in a new role as a "translator" of both medical procedures and medical language to the general public. Granted, they acknowledged, theirs may be a "weaker" vocabulary. But that was also their strength: their patients could understand them and their explanations when they sometimes felt overwhelmed by those of their physicians.[74]

The Meaning of a Nursing Identity

In early twentieth-century America, some women, if they so chose, could have a straightforward relationship with medical knowledge, expertise, and power. They could become physicians. Although more-established medical colleges remained slow to accept female students well into the twentieth century, sectarian colleges—particularly homeopathic and eclectic medical schools—proved somewhat more receptive. But as historians of women physicians have repeatedly noted, the numbers of women choosing careers as physicians began declining after 1900. The percentage of woman enrolled in medical schools, never very large in terms of absolute numbers, decreased from 5 percent in 1899, to 3.4 percent in 1905, to somewhere between 2.6 and 2.9 percent in 1910. Women were pushed from careers as physicians by gender discrimination. Still, women seemed increasingly disinclined to seek the protected niche of the homosocial institutions and discourses that had supported an earlier generation's successful storming of the male medical establishment. Indeed, as historian Regina Morantz-Sanchez argues, the early twentieth century's seemingly dispassionate and gender-neutral scientific ethos blunted support for the argument about medicine's need for the gendered perspective of a woman's sensibility and practice—in doctoring the sick.[75]

Leading nursing educators, by contrast, actively embraced a gendered perspective as they constructed a different relationship between women and medical knowledge, expertise, and power. They were less interested in storming the bastion of male medical privilege than of securing an acknowledged place within it. To this end, they simultaneously affirmed ideas about respectable womanhood and appropriated more gender-neutral representations of disciplined competence, coolness, courage, and control. They constructed their role as that of educated, supportive allies of physicians at the bedsides of sick patients. But they also saw their role as occurring in spaces where they would be the only women with the uncontested authority to engage with medical content. Nurses welcomed the military analogies because they referred not only to the male medical head but also to their own legitimate power to search for relevant pieces of medical data, to negotiate new meanings about a particular patient's symptoms, and to create new ideas about the significance of a particular clinical situation. Nursing leaders, that is, did not simply work within accepted social configurations. Rather, they deliberately manipulated carefully constructed representations to meet their own ends.

These representations, as Jennifer Fenne has argued, performed crucial ideological work. They gave nurses more power than was normally allowed women while simultaneously limiting such power by teaching nurses to also turn it inward and toward the control and discipline of themselves.[76] But these representations also held real value. They gave all nurses an identity—a persona forged out of the circumstances and experiences of learning to be a trained nurse. This identity did not depend just on the depth and breadth of medical content. This remained highly variable. Nor did it depend just on the social and racial backgrounds of those who would train as nurses. Nursing's white leadership might hope for a stage full of women like themselves. But other nurses, such as African American women like Elizabeth Jones, with whom this chapter began, could identify with the same history that made their role possible, could survive the formative processes that turned women into nurses, and could appropriate and refashion the nursing identity for the particular performances they played on their particular stages. Sometimes this came with the ironic humor that one nurse, "fresh from the farm," attached to instructions for more "lady-like ways" to haul heavy mattresses.[77] But they always came with a felt sense of place and power within their chosen field of work. They could also be critical of those who would question their background and their commitment, including those within their own ranks. "Eastern nurses," one California nurse wrote in 1912, "need to lose their prejudice of western crudeness."[78]

But if this identity was forged in training, it was deployed after graduation in communities across the nation. The manner of this deployment preoccupied the physicians who would work with such women. Each year another round of their almost formulaic graduation addresses would circulate—congratulating women on their choice of nursing as a calling, moving on to warnings of the pitfalls of pride and presumption, and concluding with an enduring portrait of the ideal nurse. T. Gaillard Thomas, a prominent white New York physician, painted his vision to a group of African American students graduating from the city's Training School for Nurses of the Colored Home and Hospital. "Let me in all seriousness sketch for you, with a pen, not a brush, the type of a model nurse," he told his audience. "She is a comely, wholesome woman," he continued, "blessed with an honest countenance, which says, as plain as a whisper in the ear, 'You can trust me.'"[79]

It seems easy to agree with educator and activist Lavinia Dock when she dismissed just such graduation addresses as "wearisome, perennial rubbish."[80] But embedded in medicine's preoccupation with character was the acknowledgement that nurses' identity also existed at the intersection of their own identities and interests. By the time Elizabeth Jones sat down to write her essay, nurses had already assumed the knowledge and the expertise needed for vigilant clinical observation and intervention: for recognizing, understanding, and responding to the meaning of discrete physiological and psychological signs and symptoms as they ebbed and flowed throughout the course of a patient's illness. They claimed, in fact, the very knowledge about practice and process that, as historian John Harley Warner has argued, was precisely what physicians—before the dawn of scientific medicine—took as their exclusive domain.[81]

The challenge to racial and gendered knowledge hierarchies was one real possibility. Thomas admonished his African American audience with a rare intensity. "When you are called upon to nurse for an obscure and unknown physician," he warned them, "beware how you presume to ignore him." This may be a physician, he acknowledged, who knew less than they did.[82] Charles V. Chapin, a longstanding supporter of nurses training schools and then superintendent of health in Providence, Rhode Island, acknowledged this in his address to the 1912 graduating class of the Butler Hospital Training School for Nurses. "It is true," he noted, "that some of our bright nurses know more about medicine than some unprogressive doctors . . . and that many of our nurses pick up some of the newer bits of knowledge which many of our physicians have yet to learn."[83] Nurses themselves knew this to be true. As one West Coast nurse wrote in jest in the *Pacific Coast Journal of Nursing:* "If a local surgeon were to ask you where you trained, tell him—with [she added] special emphasis—a New York hospital. He will be so impressed [that] he would probably ask you to do the operation."[84] Nurses' identity also existed at the intersection of the identity and interests of those who employed them. As Susan Reverby has argued, graduate nurses hired to care for a sick patients in their homes occupied an ambiguous position. They were rarely social equals at home in families' drawing rooms, nor were they servants who deserved a place in the kitchen.[85]

Still, the representations of competence, coolness, courage, and control on which nurses built their identities did create some room within which nurses could draw strength from their value and their place as they moved to assuage some or to challenge others' interests. Just as importantly, they also created an internalized and fairly stable conceptualization of "nursing" and a strong nursing identity. This identity ran across—although never bridged—the racial, gendered, and classed divide. But the early twentieth century's American educators' focus on content and character as meaningful sources of knowledge and power in the care of the sick did provide a common scaffolding upon which nurses themselves built additional meanings attendant upon their particular gendered, racialized, classed, and geographic worlds. And it encouraged nurses to consider themselves as empowered participants in the battle against disease in hospitals and homes across the country.

CHAPTER 3

They Went Nursing—in Early Twentieth-Century America

CORRINE JOHNSON KERN charmed early twentieth-century audiences with her fictional *I Go Nursing*. Her book opens at twilight in the spring of 1900 in the unnamed but easily recognizable San Francisco Hospital for Children. Kern's narrator, at seventeen, has just finished her probationary status, a short trial period before formal acceptance into nurses' training. This fictional nurse's first assignment is one she dreads with every fiber in her being. She is to care for a young child expected to die that night. "I shiver," she tells her readers, both "from cold and from fear." But she also observes. She tells her readers about breaths growing shallower and more labored as Cheyne-Stokes respirations begin to empty the lungs of the air of life. She writes of a pulse growing more and more uneven as blood struggles through the child's veins like "water through a weed-clogged stream." A door inexplicably opens, and then a floorboard creaks. "It is death," she knows, "waiting for the soul that will soon detach itself from a shrunken physical form." A hot water bottle falls to the floor, and she steadies herself lest she become completely unnerved during the child's last moments. She struggles to an open window and breathes deeply to avoid fainting. Kern's nurse turns back toward her little patient, and, as the dark of night yields to the gray of dawn, she witnesses his last convulsive quiver that sinks his body into the hollow of the bed, shrunken like a collapsed balloon. "He is dead," she says aloud although she knows there is no one to hear.[1]

This nurse's two years in training pass quickly, and in the subsequent chapters of *I Go Nursing*, readers join her on a whirlwind tour of early twentieth-century nursing practice in the western United States. Romance is, of course, threaded throughout all these stories. The narrator and a certain Dr. Karling, whose "eyes have a way of making little sparkling lights as he squints them half-closed" are deeply in love. But Kaling has left to research yellow fever in South America, risking, they both recognize, hardship and death. He writes often and sends his love. And reading and rereading his letters, the narrator admits, is often "the word that keeps me going" though the more difficult cases.[2]

Kern's nurse is as courageous as her Dr. Karling. Though terrified, she disarms a grief-stricken and crazed father who threatens her with a loaded revolver when he hears of the death of his infant son. She is also supremely competent, cool, and in absolute control of the clinical moment. She arms herself with her "implements of war"—her chart, pen, hypodermic, thermometer, cotton, and alcohol—and fights death wherever it lurks. She rescues a prostitute dying before her eyes from a typhus hemorrhage by administering a dangerous intercellular injection. She recognizes a smallpox outbreak in an isolated rural hospital near Northern Canada and immediately quarantines the institution and treats the infected lumberjacks. It is only after she uses an improvised tourniquet to save the life of a police officer shot in the line of duty that she allows herself to feel some emotions. As he smiles his gratitude while being carried to the ambulance, she horrifies herself by bursting into tears.[3]

Certainly, the experiences and attitude of Kern's nurse reflected what most people wanted in a nurse. She was competent and kind. She depended upon payments for her services to support herself, yet she also provided free care to those who could not to pay. She never refused a case although she did not like the dullness of caring for women after childbirth. She was steadfast and devoted to physicians she respected, but when she did not, she forthrightly spoke her mind and took matters into her own hands. She enjoyed the families with whom she worked yet immediately asserted her authority when they proposed their own home remedies. She sacrificed all to save her patients, and she sacrificed nothing to save her own self-respect. And her life, after her Dr. Karling returns, ends happily ever after.[4]

I Go Nursing tells a story of a life that many nurses wanted and some did experience.[5] But other trained nurses had different kinds of experiences. This chapter explores the diverse dimensions of nurses' lives in the early decades of the twentieth century. Like all women, nurses worked hard, and this chapter certainly acknowledges the sometimes problematic nature of their lives as women and as nurses in the early twentieth century. But it also uses the life stories of some of these women to explore how they understood and responded to their experiences— how they coped with the problems and exploited the opportunities that presented themselves. This chapter begins in San Francisco, at Kern's own Hospital for Children and then moves out throughout the country using both individual's stories and aggregate statistics to construct a broader and more nuanced understanding about both the work and the lives of early twentieth century nurses. In this chapter, identities forged in training confronted the realities of nursing's work. These nurses, this chapter argues, were sometimes powerful and resourceful and some- times vulnerable and alienated. But those that left detailed stories sug- gest they lead real and meaningful lives within their families, their communities, and, at times, the American health care system.

The Work and Lives of Private Duty Nurses

When Alice Burrell graduated from San Francisco's Hospital for Chil- dren Training School for Nurses in 1896, she was venturing into un- tested waters. As Mary White had earlier explained in the *Overland Monthly and Out-West Magazine,* the still "novel system of trained nursing" had only recently arrived in California.[6] The *Overland Monthly* was one voice in a chorus that championed all that would solidify San Francisco's greatness as a city as cultured and refined as any in the East. It was a city in which Frederick Law Olmsted would build a park as great as his Central Park in New York. It would have a Pacific Commercial Museum displaying the vast resources of America's new Pacific Empire much as the Philadelphia Commercial Museum highlighted those of more established trading partners.[7] And it would have a new training school for nurses that was as innovative and progressive as any in the East. The training school, White explained to her readers, was explicitly modeled after that at Bellevue Hospital in New York City, purportedly the best nurses training school in the nation. Its first director of nursing was "a quiet, composed young lady, with an intelligent, refined face . . . and a manner that would command respect in any situation" who had trained as a nurse in a leading Philadelphia hospital. The school was strongly supported by leading San Francisco citizens, including "progressive physicians" and "high class ladies."[8] Nursing as a profession was new to the West, White admitted, and the public, "unaware of its high standing in the East and abroad, as yet hardly know how to regard it." But soon, she predicted, San Francisco's trained nurses would have the same respect and standing as any nurse from Bellevue, and as many physicians, lawyers, and businessmen courting them as, she had heard, paid suit to the Bellevue graduates.[9]

The Hospital for Children's Training School was emblematic of many of the nurses training schools opening throughout the United States. It had opened in 1885 for women who would care for the little patients in the city's newest hospital while learning to become nurses.[10] But though good, it was not, like Bellevue or Johns Hopkins, among the best. Like most other American training schools, it attracted the numbers of women it needed to do the work—women like Burrell and like Kern's narrator—by sweetening the promised trade of knowledge for work with a small monthly stipend. The training school could also add the allure of being the first such school on the West Coast, but the women who entered—like most others throughout the country—were still participating in a test to find out whether their formative identities and experiences could, indeed, transform their lives.

Burrell graduated in 1896 and embarked on a peripatetic career. Her diary opens in 1899, when she is in her early 40s, in Manila, where she served for one year as a nurse with the United States Army at its 1st Reserve Hospital during the Philippine–American war.[11] She returned home to San Francisco for four months, visiting family and working nights as a private duty nurse. She then left to assume a head nurse position at the small Paia Plantation Hospital in Honolulu. Burrell stayed in that position for sixteen months, returned briefly to San Francisco, and then left immediately for New York City, where she worked as a staff nurse and a head nurse. Later, she worked as a private duty nurse for the family of Josiah Strong, a famous Protestant minister, author, and leading figure in the early twentieth-century's progressive social gospel movement. "It was one of the greatest opportunities of my life," she wrote in her diary. "They were intelligent, cultured, and *good*." She spent, in all, sixteen months in the East, moving from New York City to a postgraduate course in nursing at the Presbyterian Hospital in Chicago to a head nurse position at Grace Hospital in Detroit.[12]

In the fall of 1904, Burrell returned to San Francisco, worried about her health and a cough that did not seem to resolve. She spent one month as a patient in a sanitarium and then moved to Phoenix. The environment in Phoenix may have been better for her health but not for her career. The physicians she consulted about the possibilities of private duty practice spoke "discouragingly" about nurses' employment possibilities in that city. She returned to San Francisco in 1905 after a short sojourn as a head nurse in Los Angeles and worked as a private duty and staff nurse. But by 1908, and now in her early 50s, Burrell found fewer and fewer employment opportunities that she felt she could handle. By 1913, her health began to fail. She developed cataracts and dental problems, and she had experienced an episode of erysipelas, a painful skin infection for which she had to hire nurses to care for her. Nursing now left her back aching and her nerves "frazzled." In June of 1915 Burrell returned to San Francisco's Hospital for Children, but now as a patient and as one of a very small number of training school graduates fortunate enough to have medical costs covered by her alumnae association. Her last entry noted her hopes for a more stable teaching position with the Red Cross. Her heart condition, chronic bronchitis, enlarged gall bladder, and the "suspicious" condition of her stomach meant her private duty days were over.[13]

The outlines of Burrell's career as a trained nurse reflect what we know about private duty nursing practice. It could provide single women with exciting opportunities for work and for travel. It could also prove a stepping-stone to other kinds of work and life possibilities. Three other nurses, for example, who had also served in the Philippines and had then spent some time "bumping" around the world, decided that when they returned to California they would give up "arduous" private duty practice and open a chicken ranch. One of the three, Eugenia Venegas, told the readers of the *Overland Monthly* in 1904 that on their ranch and in their community they found respect for their nursing backgrounds, peace, independence, profit, and happy marriages to, respectively, a real estate agent, a judge, and a physician.[14] But although popular writings such as Venegas's and White's suggested that nurses might marry physicians, the reality was that some nurses *became* physicians.[15] Burrell herself considered returning to school to become an osteopathic physician, one of the easier routes women could take into medical practice.[16]

But private duty nursing practice was also fraught with problems of an already overcrowded labor market. Hundreds of trained nurses competed for limited numbers of positions in any given community. Older nurses were particularly vulnerable. Women like Burrell, worn out from and often ill because of the hard body work of sick nursing, competed with younger graduates as fresh-faced and as enthusiastic as Kern's narrator. And although Burrell had family living nearby in the Napa Valley, she, like many other trained nurses, was dependent upon herself for her own support.

But Burrell had prepared for this eventuality. Her private duty nursing practice may have been less steady than she would have preferred, but it did provide enough income to allow her to purchase two houses in San Francisco. She converted these houses to apartments, and as her nursing practice drew to a close, rental income replaced nursing wages. If she could not or would not turn to family for economic support, she did depend on them to help with other issues that would come up during her frequent absences on private duty cases. For example, she had inadvertently set fire to one of her homes while trying to test a new gas meter. Although "humiliated" that she had caused the catastrophe, she was devastated the next day when she discovered that her insurance policy had expired. On the third day, however, she was "dizzy with surprise" and deeply grateful to learn that her brother had renewed the policy during one of her absences.[17]

Other nurses' stories also suggest a sense of working as hard as one could for as long as one could and saving as much as possible for a later life of financial security. But it could be difficult for all single working women. Both Lucy Wimbash, a teacher, and her sister Emitt, a nurse, sought to provide for themselves, their mother at home in Virginia, and a future of economic independence. It was hard work. In addition to her teaching position in rural Michigan, Lucy had hoped do some sewing as a way to earn extra money. But, as she wrote her mother in 1908, "I am generally too tired after school to move or to speak."[18] Their mother missed them and often wished in her letters to them that they might miss her as much. Emitt was blunt in one reply when on duty in a Richmond, Virginia, hospital. "I don't think it is very charitable of you to wish I would get homesick when I am working and sweating like a mule."[19]

Emitt Wimbash, like Alice Burrell, carved a career in private duty out of a series of short assignments in homes, hospitals, and health care agencies. The careers of alumnae of St. Luke's Hospital Training School for Nurses in New York City suggest similar patterns.

The Women of St. Luke's

By 1938, St. Luke's Hospital, opened to treat and care for the city's Episcopalian poor, had been among the city's more prominent institutions for fifty years. Its founder, the Reverend William Augustus Muhlenberg, had created the first American Protestant nursing deaconate, the Sisterhood of the Church of the Holy Communion, to care for the hospital's patients. This deaconate was deliberately modeled on the Lutheran deaconate of Kaiserwerth, Germany—a deaconate that had yet to achieve the fame that would come when Florence Nightingale's visit there became known worldwide. It hoped to provide a life of service for devout Episcopalian women similar to that available to Roman Catholic Sisters of Charity nursing patients at New York's St. Vincent's Hospital. But the deaconate remained small, and as the St. Luke's grew in size and complexity, it moved to more secular organization of its department of nursing. It formally opened its Training School for Nurses in 1888.[20]

New York City was the center of the nursing world. It was the home of the Bellevue Hospital Training School, the country's first and still most prominent postgraduate educational program at Teachers College, and the Henry Street Settlement House, a nationally known visiting nurse service. St. Luke's quickly became one of the exemplary training schools within this realm. A member of the Vanderbilt family, long supporters of the hospital, served on the Training School's new Board of Managers. Annie Goodrich and Anna Maxwell, who would become instrumental in establishing the Army Nurse Corps, were among the prominent heads of its nursing department. Its curriculum included all the content and experiences nursing leaders believed necessary for proper training. St. Luke's Training School was among only a small number of training schools with such prestige and popularity that it demanded entrance fees rather than pay out stipends, as did Children's Hospital Training School in San Francisco, for example. As the school approached its fiftieth anniversary in 1938, its Alumnae Association decided to celebrate its accomplishments by collecting brief summaries of the work histories of its sixteen hundred graduates. It found all but thirty-six.[21]

A systematic sampling of the careers of these graduates provides one small glimpse of the life course of privileged group of early twentieth-century white nurses.[22] As at Children's, where the majority of graduates, like Burrell, remained single, most of the earliest graduates (classes of 1890 through 1899), presumably in their 60s at the time of the survey, remained unmarried (59%).[23] Most began their careers in what was then called "private duty" nursing practice, but by the late 1930s publication of their *History*, a new generation of nurses had reframed this work with the more professional term of "private nursing." These early graduates' private nursing careers remained relatively short. They worked from four to thirteen years before returning to their families. Annie Lee Pafford, for example, worked in private duty for ten years and then, like some of her single colleagues, described herself as "at home," most likely keeping house for a friend or member of her family. Those with longer careers had left nursing. Mary Louisa Jennings ('93), for example, became a physician in Geneva, New York; and Mary McVean ('94) became a tenement inspector in New York City. Like Burrell, Charlotte Shimer Hixson ('97) eventually returned to St. Luke's as a patient when seriously ill. Hixson died there as one of two graduates in this group who succumbed to the devastating 1918 influenza pandemic.[24]

The vast majority of the next generation of graduates—those graduating between 1900 and 1909—also began their careers as private nurses. A select few students were deliberately groomed for and placed in leadership positions.[25] Some 20 percent of these graduates began their careers as head nurses or supervisors responsible for the clinical education of and the care provided by younger students on hospital wards. Many of these women assumed such positions at St. Luke's. But as these particular graduates moved into their careers, the boundaries between private nursing and roles as administrators or educators became more porous. Florence Post (1908), for example, began as a private nurse and returned to St. Luke's in 1909, first as assistant head nurse, then as the head nurse of its operating rooms, until her marriage in 1918. Conversely, Ethel Stoddart (1900) worked first as a head nurse at St. Luke's before entering private practice. Others, like Elizabeth McHenry (1900), moved among different positions in New York City Hospitals and in private nursing.[26]

As with prior classes, private nursing careers of the 1900 to 1909 graduates were short. Those single women who worked for most of their lives tended to move into presumably less-taxing careers. Mary Tingle (1901), for example, spent seven of her ten years of private nursing in Paris, but upon her return the United States, she established a successful boarding house. Anna McGovern (1907) had worked as a private nurse and assistant director of nursing until, in 1920, she became a dental hygienist. Only Catherine Taylor (1902) maintained a long nursing career, but it was one well away from the stress of private and hospital practice. While she did not write classmates about her early years of practice, she described a later career in school nursing in New Mexico and California. Succeeding classes also showed increasing interest in marriage. Fifty-five percent of graduates between 1900 and 1909 had married by their 50s, and 61 percent of those graduates between 1910 and 1920 had married by their 40s.

The graduates of the classes between 1910 and 1920 provided more detailed descriptions of their work and life paths. Most worked before their marriage. But the range of work options had increased dramatically. Only 67 percent of all graduates entered private nursing upon graduation, and most of these women remained in such practice only two to three years. Many, of course, immediately answered the American and Canadian Red Cross's call for military nurses during World War I. But one-third of these St. Luke's graduates wrote of now moving directly upon graduation into roles within hospitals. This may not have been unique to graduates like those from St. Luke's. By 1924, one Children's Hospital physician regretted that too many of the hospital's graduates shunned private nursing practices for positions in hospitals. She believed its graduates feared the "new environment" they would find in their patients' homes. But her address to graduating class also suggests that the nurses themselves preferred the excitement of caring for surgical patients that they could only find in hospitals and that they also looked forward to the "executive work" that such positions also offered.[27]

Executive positions such as young head nurses or supervisors were now available. And increasingly frequent and complicated surgeries created new clinical roles for young graduates such as anesthetists and operating room "instrument passers." These clinical roles may not have been as prestigious as those in administration. Mabel Porter (1912) had to work first as an anesthetist at St. Luke's before she assumed responsibility for the operating rooms as its head nurse. But the increasing numbers of and opportunities within nursing roles in large urban hospitals like St. Luke's created the possibility of much longer careers within nursing itself. Graduates from these classes seemed to move frequently between and among positions until they finally found ones they enjoyed. Lena Wrong (1910), for example, worked for seven years as both a private nurse and a head nurse at St. Luke's until a permanent position opened up as a head nurse in its out-patient department. She remained at St. Luke's until 1921 when she accepted a position as the superintendent of the Sea Cliff Babies Convalescent Home on the New Jersey shore. She returned to St. Luke's one year later as its head admitting clerk and spent five years supervising the reams of paperwork and procedures new patients needed. In 1927, Wrong briefly served as the assistant to the head of the hospital. She retired in 1928 to a life that included some private nursing.[28]

Through the first decade of the twentieth century, a new course about "social service nursing" drew the most talented of St. Luke's students. Progressive reformers had been criticizing hospitals' increasingly reductionist and impersonal emphasis on the patient's body. The response had been an idea of a social service department that would consider that particular body as a person with real social, environmental, and economic as well as medical needs. Ideally, women in these departments would follow patients through discharge and into their homes, helping them comply with medical instructions and mobilizing necessary community resources.[29] At St. Luke's, as elsewhere, many nurses first filled this role. Indeed, as the newly professionalizing field of social work opened to women, it captured the interest of some St. Luke's nurses. Beatrice Holley (1909), for example, formally studied social work while working as an instructor of nursing first at Yale's School of Nursing and later at Bellevue's. She ultimately left nursing in 1935 to serve as a social worker in Connecticut.[30]

But St. Luke's training of students as social service nurses abruptly stopped in 1922. Even at one of the most self-consciously progressive schools of nursing, the need for students to provide all the day-to-day nursing care in the hospital limited the extent to which curricular and practice innovations could be pursued. The hospital's demands for students' work on its wards had substantively increased as it aggressively added more beds for patients and performed more complicated procedures and surgeries.[31] At St. Luke's, as in hospitals around the country, the exponentially increasing demand by hospitals for nursing students to care for its patients could not keep pace with the more slowly increasing demand of women for such positions. Many good training schools struggled during this period, and some lowered their entrance standards to attract a larger pool of candidates.

St. Luke's experience during this difficult period also suggests that a consistently strong and slowly increasing pool of well-qualified women were still choosing nursing as a career—a reality overshadowed by the surging demand. St. Luke's maintained its entrance standards and slowly increased the numbers of graduates from an average of 37 in the 1910s to 49 in the 1920s. Still, these numbers did not meet the hospital's insatiable demands. For the first time, students from training schools in specialty hospitals such as those in lying-in or psychiatric institutions were invited to work on the hospital's wards for short periods. Such "affiliations" had long been urged by leading nursing educators. They would simultaneously relieve the students of work obligations at the host institution and provide a broader range of clinical experiences to those from the affiliating ones. But affiliations were a tenuous solution. St. Luke's quickly discontinued them when the numbers of qualified applicants began more dramatically increasing in the later 1920s.[32]

Public Health Nursing

Students were denied the possibility of learning about new fields of practice by the demands of patient care. But many were then drawn, as graduates, into the expanding field of public health nursing. Public health nursing had been born in the late nineteenth-century idea of providing trained nurses to care for the country's sick immigrant and working-class families in their own homes. It had been nurtured by philanthropists who were both deeply distressed about the plight of those too poor to afford needed medical and nursing care and concerned about the threats of infection that the untreated germs of these same men, women, and children posed to them, to their families, and to their communities. It had come of age when talented and ambitious nurses seized opportunities to constantly demonstrate how intensive nursing care saved lives and prevented the spread of infectious illnesses.

The nurses at New York City's Henry Street Settlement House played a critical role in the development of this new field of nursing practice. Henry Street was founded and led by Lillian Wald, a New York Hospital Training School graduate who had left medical school when she felt she could do more for immigrant families in the city's lower east side by practicing as a nurse rather than as a physician. It was supported by prominent New York businessmen and women. Through the opening decades of the twentieth century, it could point to a string of stunning successes. In 1902, for example, Wald had persuaded the city's public school system to allow a Henry Street nurse to care for students who had been sent home with suspected infectious diseases; this nurse would make sure that the children received proper care and that their families learned how to prevent further infections. By 1909, what had begun as a "demonstration project" involved more than 140 newly titled "school nurses" working with sick school children and their families as employees of the city's Board of Health.[33] At the same time, Wald had promised executives from the Metropolitan Life Insurance Company (MLI) that they would pay substantially fewer death benefits to the families of its policyholders if they provided them with a Henry Street nurse to care for them when sick. By 1911, given the plummeting death rates that accompanied such nursing care, MLI was providing this benefit to policyholders across the nation, and by 1914 it was paying for over one million visits by trained nurses to its sick policyholders.[34]

Some St. Luke's graduates worked for Henry Street. Margaret Reid (1920), for example, first gained experience as a private and hospital nurse before joining the Settlement House in 1922. She enjoyed a long career as a public health nurse with the American Red Cross and, finally, as the director of nursing education at MLI.[35] The impetus behind institutions like Henry Street and practices like public health nursing was repeating itself, albeit less dramatically, in urban communities across the country. More and more, St. Luke's training school graduates were describing their work with public health departments as school nurses ensuring the health of children, with charity organizations as visiting nurses caring for the sick poor in their own homes, and with private tuberculosis associations as nurses committed to finding, treating, and educating patients and their families as part of a national campaign to eradicate this disease.

Octavia Briggs, Alice Burrell's classmate in the 1896 graduating class of the Children's Hospital Training School, had established San Francisco's first nurses' settlement house with three colleagues in 1898.[36] Like its eastern counterpart, the Tehama Street Settlement House provided valuable care and assistance to the city's immigrants and white working families through its nurses. But it largely ignored, as did many other civic organizations, the health and illness needs of the city's large Chinese population. This racial discounting cast into sharp relief what historians have described as a political subtext to the work of public health nurses. As historian Karen Buhler-Wilkerson has argued, these women brought "medicine and a message" into the homes they visited. They provided critically important services while delivering them in a context that taught American standards and middle-class values to soon-to-be citizens and to the aspiring poor.[37] In early twentieth-century America, however, Chinese men and women—no matter that they may have been born in the United States—were denied the right to ever earn citizenship. There was little need to teach them the norms of white America. Protestant missionary organizations like the one that hired nurse Harriet Phillips saw to their health and welfare needs.[38]

With the needs of so many of its inhabitants so invisible, public health nursing in San Francisco grew at a much slower rate than in eastern and midwestern cities. The absolute numbers also remained small. Yssabella Waters' 1905 survey, for example, counted twenty-nine such nurses in New York City and sixteen in San Francisco.[39] Her later 1909 survey, however, counted hundreds in New York City, many working for the city's health department as school nurses. San Francisco, by contrast, had fifteen—about half the rate of public health nurse per person as New York City—working in schools or with one or two other colleagues in tuberculosis identification and prevention campaigns and in the homes of the sick poor and immigrants.[40] By 1916 San Francisco counted fewer than thirty such nurses, including two who now worked in department stores providing emergency first aid.[41]

The numbers of public health nurses grew steadily as the federal government, through the Sheppard-Towner legislation of the early 1920s, provided funds to send such nurses into communities across the country to teach new mothers about the importance of proper infant feeding and child care in the fight against infant mortality. This important work was not necessarily glamorous. In the seven months she had worked as a public health nurse for one California county, Sophia Balch wrote in 1921, "it's been bumping along over country roads, stopping at schools—sometimes all day, sometimes only for an hour or two, for physical exams and for home visits afterwards. Then, of course, there have been communicable disease investigation and T.B. work, considerable social service, *and many* conferences with folks, that are intended to educate the public."[42]

The idea and the practice of public health nursing had an enormous impact on nursing education. Given the unwillingness of even progressive schools like St. Luke's to teach about the social needs of patients or the principles of good health and health teaching, new postgraduate training opportunities had to be established. Not surprisingly, New York City led the way when the prominent philanthropist, Teachers College trustee and Wald supporter Helen Hartley Jenkins created an endowment in 1909 to establish what was announced with great fanfare in the *New York Times* as a "post graduate course for teacher nurses, who will carry the theory and practice of hygienic living into schools, houses, factories, stores, and communities" at Teachers College.[43] Formal postgraduate training quickly became courses that provided college credits. Series of courses quickly became programs that awarded baccalaureate degrees in nursing education, administration, or public health. The groundwork had been laid for loosening the grip of hospital training schools.

By 1921, San Francisco had its own opportunities for nursing education similar to that available in other large northern cities. Young San Franciscan women who would nurse might, if they so chose, attend Stanford University. After two years of hospital training in Stanford's hospital in San Francisco and an additional three years of education on its Palo Alto campus, nurses would graduate with a baccalaureate degree. They would be not only "competent nurses" but also nurses equipped through special training "for responsible positions as administrators, teachers, and supervisors in hospitals and in nurses training schools, and for community service work along the lines of public health and social service."[44] Those who had already earned their hospital diplomas had another option. They might choose instead to attend summer school at the University of California and, though courses such as "Bacteriology," "Child Welfare," "Principles of Public Health Nursing," and "Field Work," slowly build their credits toward an eventual college degree.[45]

The Life and Work of One Public Health Nurse

Isabel Glover's unfinished autobiography, written after she had retired to San Francisco in 1945, provides a glimpse into how the possibilities, the problems, and the politics of public health nursing practice played themselves out in women's lives. Glover, born and reared on the plains of Nebraska, began her career, like her mother, as a teacher. However, she hated teaching. She had problems disciplining her students, and after three years in three different teaching positions, she felt like a "total failure." She attended the Nebraska Normal School for Teachers hoping to improve her skills, but by the early 1910s, she felt her career had hit a dead end. She found herself teaching in the same school she had attended as a child and with a social life, she noted with some irony, whose highlight was attending the annual state teachers' conference.[46]

Roy Eaton, her brother's friend, came into her life in 1913, and by 1914 they were engaged to be married. Glover felt transformed: that magic word "engaged," she remembered, "changed my whole attitude toward physical contact." As she planned her wedding ceremony, she accepted a teaching position in rural Montana near the Canadian border where Eaton worked in her brother's lumber business. She felt miserable, isolated, and scared of the possibility of her helplessness should she become ill. Glover knew of other women who had enjoyed attending nursing school at the University of Colorado's hospital in Boulder. She broke her engagement to Eaton and entered training, fully aware that she had always avoided being with friends when they were sick and gratefully assured by hospital that she would be under no obligation to stay if she did not like it.[47]

To her surprise, Glover loved her training school experience. "It had felt," she remembered, "almost as if I was on the outside of life and now

I was on the inside." Despite its prestigious sounding name, the Hospital of the University of Colorado was, in fact, a 40-bed hospital that primarily treated sick and injured miners. It did not meet national nursing standards, but it did offer its students the opportunity to take courses for credit at the University, and its curriculum included one lecture on public health nursing. That one lecture, with its discussion of the Henry Street Settlement and Teachers College, Glover wrote, "opened a whole world of new possibilities." She had met Andrew Bachels when she was a junior, working twelve-hour shifts, and taking a university course on European history. He had been hospitalized when he became sick with measles and pneumonia during a trip to Boulder. But, although tempted, she refused to consider his romantic advances. He was fourteen years older that she was, and he was a Catholic, while she was a devout Presbyterian. But the most important reason the relationship could not continue, she told him, was that she had discovered public health nursing, and "that was enough to interest me for the rest of my life."[48]

But Glover first needed money to realize her ambition. She enlisted in the army through the American Red Cross upon her graduation in 1917 and spent a year nursing soldiers at Camp Logan in Texas.[49] After the war, she won a Red Cross scholarship to Teachers College that included a period of preliminary field work with the prominent Chicago Visiting Nurse Association (VNA). Within the small world of public health nursing, relationships could be personal and intimate. Edna Foley, the nationally known director of this VNA, took Glover under her wing and slowly introduced her to the realities of poor, urban life.[50] Foley assigned Glover to the immigrant Hull House district on Chicago's south side. It was, she remembered, her first introduction to the inequities in American life. "It would not take many years in a big city," she wrote her mother in 1919, "to make me a rank socialist or something worse." The presumption that it was only the "generosity of the rich" that enabled the poor to receive nursing care, she continued, "makes my blood boil."[51]

It was in Chicago that Glover first confronted her own feelings about race. Large, northern and urban public health nursing groups like the VNA in Chicago and Henry Street had always been among the most progressive organizations within nursing. They had a longstanding commitment to providing care across the color line, and many had as long a history of hiring talented African American nurses. There were limits to their progressivism, however. Those that hired African American nurses assigned them to care only for African American patients. There was only occasionally equitable pay and working conditions and almost no opportunity for advancement into supervisory positions.[52] For a woman like Glover, who never had to think about her feelings about race relations because she had never worked with someone from a different racial background, working on relatively equal terms with African American colleagues was a profound experience. Her admitted unease when one sat next to her on a streetcar forced her to confront the fact that she too could harbor a "germ" of prejudice.[53]

Glover's experience at Teachers College was remembered as a whirl of experiences: living with students from all over the country, dining with Adelaide Nutting, volunteering at Henry Street, and taking in the sights and sounds of New York City. It was also the place that nurtured her ambition of starting a formal public health nursing program in Boulder. Nutting urged her to be cautious: she had heard that the University of Colorado had plans for a public health nursing course but that the content of that course was not "constructive" university-level work. Once back in Boulder in 1920, Glover agreed that the prospect for public health nursing seemed "not very promising." She resigned from her first position in the city's health department when a promised raise did not come through, and in a small nursing world where connections remained important, Foley helped her obtain a one-year position with an Indianapolis public health nursing association, teaching nursing students about public health nursing.[54]

However much Glover may have loved public health nursing, she was temperamentally unsuited for its practice and politics. Indianapolis refused to renew her contract: her paperwork was disorganized, she could not effectively organize the work that needed to be done each day, and her relationships with co-workers had deteriorated to the point where they had made it clear to her that she did not belong in that agency. Glover appealed to Foley for help—but now Foley refused. Foley had presumably heard about her problematic tenure. There were issues, she wrote back to her, that she "needed to face squarely" if she were to be successful in public health nursing practice. These issues centered on the heart of public health nursing practice. They were not ones of deference to physicians; they involved collaboration both with patients and with her peers. Did her patients, Foley wondered, look forward to her visits? Did the students who worked for her approach her with respect and affection as well as obedience? And did her nursing colleagues and supervisors feel they could approach her honestly and openly with criticism as well as with praise?[55]

Glover entered what she later described as "the most frustrating experience of my life." Her connections again helped. A fellow Teachers College graduate was able to get her a public health nursing position in rural Vermilion County in western Indiana as she thought about her future and Foley's questions. Eighteen months later, in March of 1924, she again wrote to Foley, thanking her for her honesty and admitting "that no amount of kindness would have put me on my feet." She impressed Foley with both her reflectiveness and the changes she had made in her practice. In her letter back to Glover, Foley noted that "she had rarely received such a positive response to criticism." And later, when the position of director of public health nursing opened at the Indiana State Board of Health, Foley recommended her.[56]

This would be a position of power and responsibility for Glover. She would travel throughout the state, persuading local communities who preferred to hire their own community's hospital trained nurses as their public health nurses that they should, instead, hire outsiders who were specifically educated for public health nursing practice. She would be politically sensitive, careful never to recommend a Catholic public health nurse in a state known as a seat of Klan activity. But Glover had no sooner begun this position when a persistent cough led to a diagnosis of "minimal tuberculosis." Glover had resources: the state of Indiana provided a three-month leave with full pay while she sought treatment; and her earlier service in the army entitled her to receive treatment at a Veterans Hospital near her family in Colorado. But she also lost her position. Her assistant, she steadfastly believed, constantly undercut her and her initiatives during her absence.[57]

Glover's family helped her through this trying time. By 1928, she felt well enough to do what many nurses with a history of tuberculosis did: she assumed a part-time position working in the field as a tuberculosis nurse in Denver.[58] By 1930, she had finally agreed to marry Andrew Bachels. They had kept in contact over the years and had rekindled their romance in 1929 when he met her in California at a national tuberculosis conference she attended. Within a few short years she found herself poor, pregnant, and isolated at her new husband's Canadian mine. Her husband had lost his $25,000 savings in the stock market crash, and his mine was no longer productive. Her pregnancy was at risk because of her age—she was in her early 40s—and her history of tuberculosis. Her nearest female neighbor happened to be a private duty nurse with whom she felt she had little in common. Glover, with her husband and their new baby, left the mine in the early 1930s and entered what she later remembered as the "most difficult" of all the years of her life.[59]

The Depression of the 1930s hit most nurses hard. Certainly some, like Daisy Barnwell Jones, had husbands with secure government positions and practices with rich and powerful patients.[60] But most, like Glover, struggled as patients' demand for private nursing plummeted and both hospitals and public and private health care agencies eliminated expensive positions. The situation was so desperate among nurses that Franklin Roosevelt's New Deal had its own Works Project Administration program aimed at providing them with some small employment possibilities as public health nurses in communities across the nation. Other federal agencies offered a few other possibilities. Glover accepted a position with the National Bureau of Maternal and Child Health that offered four months work each year in the mountains of northwest California. She wanted and needed this position and promised herself that she would not get involved in any patronage controversies. She did not, but she was promptly fired when she refused to stop teaching school children about masturbation. Glover and her family were not completely destitute, however. Her husband had some small bond income, and he later qualified for Social Security payments. She eventually renewed her teaching certificate and spent the waning years of the Depression in San Francisco accepting intermittent teaching and nursing positions.[61] Glover joined many other nurses, moving by choice, by chance, or by circumstances between nursing and other kinds of work options.

The Women of Lincoln

The stories of African American nurses who trained at New York City's Lincoln Hospital School of Nursing tell of similar kinds of movements.

Lincoln Hospital existed within the segregated system of health and illness care in the United States. It had been established and run by philanthropic white women as first a home and later a hospital for elderly and chronically ill African American men and women. The hospital had opened its nurses training school in 1898 with white nursing superintendents teaching and supervising the work of African American students. By the early 1920s, in a new location in the city's South Bronx, it drew many of its neighborhood's poor, white, and chronically ill residents who had their own separate physical space within the hospital. These particular white patients did not object to receiving nursing care by African American women. This work existed within traditions of slavery and service. They did object to receiving medical care by African American men, however. This work existed within knowledge and power hierarchies that would, if allowed, invert the norms of white supremacy, and it invoked white suspicions of African American men's sexual intent with white women patients. The hospital had no African American medical attending or student staff.[62]

By the early 1930s, the Lincoln Hospital School of Nursing had its own endowment, a city-supported mission to extend care to all poor African Americans, and a reputation—shared by both white philanthropists and African American nurses—as one of the best training schools in the country for African American women.[63] Teachers College white nursing faculty, surveying the school at its own request in 1931, considered the school "outstanding." The survey, however, acknowledged substantial problems. The deteriorating condition of both the hospital and its nurses' home contributed to a rate of student illnesses twice that of those nursing students who lived and worked in the newer buildings at the city's Harlem Hospital, New York City's other African American hospital. Moreover, Lincoln's students had higher failure rates on the state registration exams than those of white peers.[64]

The Teachers College survey also acknowledged problems at Lincoln that plagued many white training schools throughout the country. Many Lincoln students provided thoughtful and careful care. But many found themselves assigned responsibilities for which they were completely unprepared and for which they had little ward teaching or supervision by more experienced students or head nurses. The survey commended the school for its ambitious agenda of remaining aligned with the goals of the most progressive schools of nursing in the country. It did, however, concur with the racist limits surrounding Lincoln's dreams for its future. Lincoln might be the best African American school of nursing in the country, but its ambition, the survey noted, could only take it to a place among the "better" of white American training schools.[65]

The community respected Lincoln graduate nurses. Physicians who worked with them believed their work comparable to that of white nurses with whom they also worked. But the work options of these women were sharply curtailed by northern social norms and racial practices. A Lincoln graduate who wished to work as a private nurse could only do so in African American families, in white families who also employed African Americans in other positions, or in hospitals with an African American training school. The critical issue involved meals. African Americans in the North might eat in the same public dining room as white men and women, but they could not eat in the same space with them in a private home.[66] Mary Mahoney, often cited as the first African American trained nurse, acknowledged that these kinds of racial norms affected her practice in Massachusetts. White colleagues, when nursing within a private home, could ask for a separate meal to be served them in their patient's room. She had to take her meals in the family's kitchen. Mahoney, however, maintained the status of her position by demanding that she eat alone in the family's kitchen at a time other than when the servants ate.[67]

Moreover, a Lincoln graduate who wished to work as a public health nurse or in a hospital had to compete for a limited number of employment possibilities. The only positions available were in large public health agencies or hospitals that served enough African American patients to justify hiring an African American nurse who would care only for them. Many such graduates found themselves as the first African Americans to work for their particular agencies. For example, Marguerite Harris, a 1925 graduate, worked as the first African American hired by the Patterson, New Jersey, Department of Public Health. She also went on to become the first African American nurse to earn a baccalaureate degree in nursing from Seton Hall University.[68] But nurses like Harris could never advance from staff to supervisory positions. An African American nurse could never stand in judgment of the work of a white colleague.

Even at Lincoln, the prerogatives of whiteness took precedence over class, education, and training. The hospital's white administration refused to formally appoint an African American nurse as the director of nursing, even though Adah Thoms, a Richmond-educated teacher and a 1905 graduate of Lincoln, ran the school. During her tenure, Thoms instituted a postgraduate certificate program for African American nurses who needed to broaden their clinical experiences. Graduates of this postgraduate program provided the backbone of African American nursing leadership and included Martha Minerva Franklin, a Woman's Hospital of Philadelphia Training School graduate who joined Mahoney and Thoms in establishing the first African American nursing organization, the National Association of Colored Graduate Nurses. They also included Hulda Margaret Lyttle, who had graduated from Nashville's George W. Hubbard Training School for Nurses in 1914 and who later assumed a prominent leadership position among African American nurses as the superintendent of nurses at Meharry Medical College School of Nursing in Nashville, Tennessee. Thoms also worked to convince the American Red Cross to accept a limited number of African American nurses into the armed services during World War I. Yet despite her accomplishments, her formal title at Lincoln was always that of "acting" director of nursing, a title she held until her retirement in 1923.[69]

In the main, the Teachers College survey correctly noted, the significant contributions of African American nurses were "confined to members of their own race because of race prejudices." Even in situations within their own race, "many professional opportunities are closed to them." Not surprisingly, given the limited employment possibilities, many such women did not remain in nursing. In preparation for an alumnae report that would be part of the Teachers College survey, Lincoln could only locate 58 percent of its graduates, and the Teachers College questionnaire subsequently sent to these 254 nurses yielded only 81 responses. Those who responded had relatively stable paid employment. The majority of them had positions as public health nurses, and 25 percent had positions in institutions. Less than 20 percent confronted the instability of private nursing practice. They had come to Lincoln from areas across the United States, but few returned home. Of these, 72 percent remained in New York City, and another 10 percent remained in the surrounding geographical area. Few settled in the southern United States. As the report aptly stated, "Nurses who have been educated in Northern cities are not inclined to accept the less favorable social and economic conditions of southern communities."[70]

Granted, there is little indication that Lincoln alumnae had the time or the resources that their white peers at St. Luke's had to doggedly track down almost every single graduate. But the low response rate also suggests a sense that many such graduates had moved on to other opportunities with their lives and careers. Many, if not most, were pushed out of careers they wanted by poor employment prospects. But some had moved on to others. Nella Larsen, a 1915 graduate, was traveling through France at the time of the survey as the first African American woman to win a coveted and prestigious Guggenheim Fellowship to study abroad.

Nella Larsen: One Story of Identity and Work

Nella Larsen's life path provides one stunning example of the range of possibilities nursing offered to talented and ambitious women. She was born in 1891 to immigrant parents: her white mother was from Denmark, and her black father was from the Danish West Indies. Larsen never knew her father, and after her mother married, she grew up with a white step-father and half-sister. Larsen's mother, keenly aware that her black daughter would have fewer opportunities for meaningful work than her white one, believed education was the key to Larsen's future. In 1907 she sent her to Fisk University, one of the most prestigious African American colleges, to train as a teacher. Larsen did not last long at Fisk. She chafed against the university's discipline and the strict dress code it had established as a signifier of the virtue and the protected morality of the young and single African American women who lived and learned there side by side with young men. Fisk asked that she leave after one year.

Larsen spent some years in her mother's homeland and, in 1912, moved to New York City. As her biographer, George Hutchinson, points out, Larsen quickly found herself particularly vulnerable to the racialized structure of a labor market that welcomed African American women as domestic servants but had few places for those who wanted work that drew on their education.[71] Nursing offered one respectable option for support during the process of learning about the work. Larsen enrolled in the Lincoln Hospital School of Nursing in 1912. Adah Thoms recognized her talent, developed her skills, and, upon her graduation in 1915, arranged a prestigious position for Larsen as a head nurse at the Tuskegee Institute's John A. Andrew Memorial Hospital, an African American hospital in one of the country's best-known African American institutions. Booker T. Washington, the founder of the Tuskegee Institute, had died by the time Larsen arrived at the Alabama hospital, but his commitment to teaching and nursing as instrumental in African American women's social and economic self-help crusade remained strong.

Larsen, however, disliked the hospital and hated the South. Within one year, she had returned to New York City and to a position as Thoms' assistant at Lincoln. Like many talented nurses, Larsen moved quickly into public health—and a much-sought-after civil service position in the city's health department. Her personal life flourished alongside her professional one. She met and married the African American physicist Elmer Imes and, through him, moved into the world of the city's intellectual elite at the dawn of the Harlem Renaissance. Their friends included such African American luminaries as Walter White, the activist head of New York's chapter of the National Association for the Advancement of Colored People. They also included James Weldon Johnson, a lawyer, composer and author, with his brother, J. Rosamond Johnson, of "Lift Ev'ry Voice and Sing," soon to be adopted by the NAACP as the "Negro National Anthem." Their friendships crossed the color line. They remained close to Carl Van Vechten, a white novelist and supporter of African American authors, even after his own book, *Nigger Heaven,* split the African American literary community. *Nigger Heaven,* an allusion to the balconies in movie theaters where Northern Jim Crow segregated their African American audiences, purported to make the "great black walled city" of Harlem visible to white America. Langston Hughes, like Larsen, liked the book. Others, like W.E.B. DuBois, saw it as an affront.

Van Vechten had long encouraged Larsen to pursue her own literary ambitions. Larsen moved slowly at first, continuing to work as a nurse after her marriage while writing children's stories and volunteering at the 135th Street Branch of the New York Public Library, an emerging center of African American intellectual life. In 1923 she decided to leave nursing and become a librarian. Her literary life then moved more quickly. By 1928, with the publication of her first novel, *Quicksand,* to wide critical acclaim, she had resigned her position as a librarian and emerged as one of the most celebrated novelists of the Harlem Renaissance.

Heady years followed. In 1929, she published *Passing* to equal acclaim. In 1930, she traveled through France and Spain on her Guggenheim Fellowship. Then Larsen's world crashed. Accusations of plagiarism surrounded her short story "Sanctuary." She learned of her husband's longstanding affair with a white administrator at Fisk University. Her publisher rejected her third book manuscript. She began struggling with alcohol abuse. Larsen and Imes formally divorced in 1937. A generous alimony settlement provided her with financial security. It also allowed her to slip into the life of a recluse as she deliberately withdrew from her longstanding circle of friends.

Imes's death in 1940 shattered the protective shell within which Larsen lived. By 1944, with no more alimony, she again needed to support herself. She returned to nursing—much to the chagrin of a later generation of literary scholars who have cast her return to her original life's work as a "surrender," a "disappearance," an act of self-burial, or a "retreat" motivated by a lack of courage and dedication. Her most recent biographer has challenged these interpretations as only reflective of the attitudes of those who looked down upon or did not understand the work and worth of nursing.[72] Larsen, in fact, used nursing to reconstruct a quieter, more stable, perhaps less exciting, although no less important life as an effective and respected hospital nursing administrator until her death in 1964.

Nella Larsen's voice remains strong in her books still in print and in her re-emerging literary reputation as one of the most significant authors of the early twentieth-century Harlem Renaissance. Her voice speaks to the complexity of identities and to the real complications that sometimes confine and sometimes frustrate black women's search for a secure footing. Her characters stand at the crossroads of gender, race, and class. They experience a world of profound ambiguities. And they constantly explore, sometimes successfully, and sometimes unsuccessfully, the kinds of recreated identities that might bring them a sense of peace if not always one of fulfillment.

The voices heard in the novels, diaries, letters, and survey responses of women who worked as nurses might also be considered as emblematic of Larsen's experience. Upon graduation, these women too entered an ambiguous and uncertain world. As they made their way through this world, some found that their hard work compromised their health and sense of well-being. Others found moments of satisfaction that transcended their sense of self. Some white nurses experienced sheer frustration with the prospects of little work and no money. Other African American nurses experienced sheer frustration with the racial practices that guaranteed little work and no money. Some nurses found safety in the relationships and networks that helped them through their careers. Others found that competition led them to choose other work. These nurses had much in common with Larsen's characters. All constantly explored other ways of recreating their lives—both within and outside nursing. In this they were not unsuccessful. Their enduring sense of themselves as competent, courageous, and controlled opened all kinds of possibilities.

CHAPTER 4

Wives, Mothers—and Nurses

IN 1924, MARIA JOHNSON traveled from her native Salt Lake City, Utah, for New York City and its prestigious baccalaureate program in public health nursing at Columbia University's Teachers College. Johnson was the well-educated granddaughter of two Mormon pioneers. She had worked first as a teacher before following a cherished desire to enter nursing. She had graduated from Latter-Day Saints (LDS) Hospital Training School for Nurses in Salt Lake City in 1919 and then worked briefly as a surgical nursing supervisor at the LDS Hospital and as a school nurse in Utah's rural counties.[1]

Johnson was a faithful church member and an ambitious nurse. With her new baccalaureate degree from Teachers College in hand, she left New York City in 1926 for a position as the field representative of the American Red Cross in San Francisco. Six years later she returned Utah and to her training school alma mater as its superintendent of nurses and director of its newly renamed School of Nursing. She successfully led the LDS Hospital School of Nursing for sixteen years. At a time when most schools of nursing throughout the country remained wedded to a hospital-based nurses training program, Johnson negotiated a collegiate affiliation with the University of Utah that made it easier for her students to further their education. She shepherded her school through successful accreditation processes by the National League for Nursing Education, an organization whose voluntary educational standards went well beyond those required by the state. Johnson solidified the school's reputation as the flagship school in the expanding LDS Hospital system in the intermountain West and as one of the best in the state.

In 1938 the Salt Lake City radio station KSL recognized Johnson's achievements in a program focusing on outstanding Utah women. By the time she retired in 1946, Johnson held a place among the small but influential group of American nursing leaders. She had served on state committees addressing mobilization and distribution of nurses during World War II and had held prominent positions on the boards of state and national nursing associations. Marie Johnson died in 1974 at the age of eighty-six.[2] She would be remembered as "the dean of Utah nursing."[3] Her nursing colleagues paid her their highest tribute. She was, they remembered, "a nurse's nurse, a doctor's nurse, and a patient's nurse."[4]

Maria Johnson's story of prominence and achievement was one kind of life lived as a nurse. Roxana Farnsworth Hase, Johnson's fellow 1919 LDS Hospital Nurses Training School graduate, has provided examples of many others as well. Hase collected the life stories of the training school's graduates when the LDS Hospital School of Nursing Alumnae Association sought data for the school's 50th anniversary celebration in 1955. Hase paid particular attention to gathering the stories of her own classmates and succeeded in collecting the life stories of all seventeen of her fellow graduates. These stories provide a rare collective biography, of sorts, that shows the enormous range with which one group of white women, united only by a training school experience, interpreted notions of what work meant over almost six decades of their lives.

These stories, enriched with genealogical data from the LDS Family History Library, allow a look back to two generations and forward to more than sixty years of lives as wives, mothers, and nurses. They, and those of other LDS Hospital Training School graduates, give us another way to think more deeply and more contextually about the meaning of identity and work for nurses in particular and for women in general. These stories tell of women who always worked. But over the course of a lifetime, much of the work took place, not just within hospitals and health care agencies, where we have traditionally placed it. Their work also took place within their families and within their families' particular patterns of wage work and unremunerated housework, care work, and work on farms or small businesses. In their life stories we see how these women, either by choice or by circumstances, moved rather easily and intermittently back and forth between home and hospital and between the domestic and market economies. Their paid work was not separate from their work as wives and mothers. It was instead deeply integrated.

The graduates of LDS Training School class of 1919 do not stand for any typical trained nurse. These women lived and worked as white

Mormon women, deeply embedded in an explicitly hierarchical and patriarchal religious tradition that privileged motherhood and women's domestic responsibilities over that of paid work.[5] They were raised within the familial, social, and religious norms of the Church of Jesus Christ of Latter-day Saints (LDS), and many remained faithful to such norms for their entire lives. But their richly described life stories and those of other graduates do illustrate one way in which nursing stood at the nexus of powerful ideas about women, work, family, and religion. In these stories, as this chapter argues, we can see how within the world of early twentieth-century Mormon Utah, nursing represented an opportunity for women to construct lives that held significant and socially legitimate options within their fairly conservative structural place.

For these women, the value of nursing's care work was not solely measured in terms of ideas, identities, or the possibilities of the wage labor market. It was also measured by its meaning. Nursing represented a way that Mormon women might remain active and empowered participants in constructing meaningful lives, in supporting their families' domestic economy, and in participating in their communities' social world. It gave these women a range of choices at particular moments in historical time, over the course of their family's life cycle, and through the unpredictability of life events and changing aspirations. And it emphasized the ability of private rather than public strategies that helped women reconcile the demands of work and family life. In twentieth-century Mormon Utah, then, nursing work presented an opportunity, albeit no promise, for particular women with relatively limited means but considerable ambition to reach for the stars with both feet planted firmly on earth.

A Changing World

The seventeen graduates of the LDS Hospital Training School Class of 1919 were all born into the Church of Jesus Christ of Latter-day Saints. The LDS Church, like so many other Protestant denominations, emerged from the swirl of social and religious revivalism that swept upstate New York in the early nineteenth century. In its doctrines and practices, however, it quickly became one of the most conservative, controversial, and even despised of all those in nineteenth-century America. Antipathy drew from many sources. The lower-class backgrounds of many of the American and British Mormon converts persuaded onlookers that only the most dispossessed and distasteful could hold such peculiar beliefs as a divinely revealed Book of Mormon and the divinely ordered practice of polygamy. The Mormon commitment to a literal restoration of the kingdom of God convinced others that their ultimate allegiance was to their church rather than to their country.

More pragmatically, Mormon settlements threatened the political and economic viability of previously established communities. Their collective vision meant they would only do business with each other, they would vote as a political block, they would assert their God-given as well as their legal right to land, and they would maintain their own armed militia. Their growing numbers turned this threatened power into a reality.[6] After deadly battles in settlements in Ohio and Missouri, Mormons recognized that they would have to move.[7] Between 1846 and 1887, more than 85,000 Mormons from America and Europe, along with an uncounted number of their children, moved to the Utah territory. According to historian H. H. Bancroft, it was a "migration without parallel in the world's history."[8]

The charismatic Brigham Young led the Mormons as they built a society in what they believed to be the glorious isolation of the Utah desert. There the LDS Church determined the curriculum of territorial schools and owned and operated businesses, factories, and mining companies. Church directives dominated Utah politics, and LDS Church members invariably held the key positions in the territorial administrative structure. The social structure of the church replicated that of its families. The LDS men's priestly powers to act in God's name would be definitive, and virtually all Mormon men over the age of twelve could be priests.[9] Mormon women acted through the church's Relief Society, the female counterpart, companion, and complement to the LDS men's priesthood.[10] The women's Relief Society was responsible for the health, education, and the social and economic self-sufficiency of the thousands of Mormon women and children settling the Utah territory. Its structure supported women's sharing with men the performance of formal healing rituals that called upon the power of prayer to comfort and cure.[11]

The self-sufficiency and isolation sought by Mormons proved elusive, however. The last golden spike in a new transcontinental railroad was driven into the ground at Promontory Summit just north of Salt Lake

City in 1869, and the railroad subsequently brought thousands of non-believing emigrants to the territory. The invention of dynamite, mechanized drills, and technologically efficient smelters brought numerous national and international investors to Utah's mineral mines as well as European and Chinese immigrants seeking work in them. Furthermore, mainstream America, fresh from its abolition of southern slavery, renewed its fight to eliminate polygamy—now seen as the last problematic source of substantive political, social, and economic subversion.[12] After a long struggle, an 1887 federal law criminalized polygamy, confiscated most LDS Church property, disbanded Utah's militia, and took control of the territory's educational system. Finally, in 1890, LDS Church leaders formally renounced polygamy and set about establishing a new order that would preserve essential religious doctrines, provide enough political influence to protect the interests of the church, and allow the Mormons increased tolerance and acceptance by mainstream American society.[13]

As the LDS Church moved to create new paths through the thickets of demands placed on it when it renounced polygamy and increased its involvement in the secular world, it drew its members into more defined and more protected religious and social spaces. The 1919 LDS nursing school graduates came of age as their church strengthened its organizational hierarchy, centralized administrative structures, and reemphasized the authority of its male priesthood.[14] The women in the Relief Society were no longer to see themselves as a complement to the men's priesthood. They were now to be but one of a number of other organizations functioning under priesthood direction.[15] Marriage and motherhood remained, for Mormon women, a sacred and eternal calling. But unlike plural wives who won praise for their economic support of extended families, early twentieth-century Mormon women were now warned of the "dangerous power" of an independently earned income.[16] Moreover, their role in religious healing and care belonged to their past. "Any good sister," the LDS Church presidency wrote to members of the Relief Society in 1914, "full of faith in God and in the efficacy of prayer," could still anoint the sick with oil.[17] However, Mormon women lost their formal authority to "seal" their blessings on their sick. That would now the prerogative of a more influential, and more institutionalized, men's priesthood.[18]

At the same time, Utah itself was looking less like God's kingdom and more and more like mainstream American society. By 1890 more than

44 percent of Utah's population was non-Mormon. While Utah remained the domain of small family farms, its population centers were tilting toward the cities. In fact, when Utah became the nation's forty-fifth state in 1896, its relative proportion of urban to rural residents mirrored that of the country as a whole. Meanwhile, industrialization was exploding, spurred on by new strip mining technologies in the copper and coal industries. The mining industry's insatiable demand for labor, in turn, fueled a new move now of Greek, Italian, and southern Slavic immigrants to the state, where they joined a much smaller community of African Americans who worked as porters for the railroad companies. Religious visions of homogeneous, self-sufficient communities working for the collective good were, in fact, rather smoothly giving way to communities that were more individualistic, increasingly entrepreneurial, and market driven.[19]

Even Salt Lake City, the historic heart of the LDS Church's administrative and religious network, was fast shedding its exclusively Mormon identity. It was now the heart of the rapidly expanding mining, railroad, manufacturing, commercial, and financial industries whose demand for labor fueled a more secularized population growth from 12,000 inhabitants in 1870 to just over 58,000 in 1890.[20] The city's census grew again to 77,000 in 1900 as it recovered from the depression of the 1890s and then almost doubled to 131,000 by 1910.[21] Salt Lake City, like so many other American cities, was fast becoming a place of great wealth and great poverty. But through all these changes, the city's Mormon and non-Mormon leadership joined in a commitment to the civic virtues of a market-driven economy and the social virtues of self-reliance and self-sufficiency.[22] Efficiency, administration, and infrastructure were the domain of city governance; education, social service, and relief would be that of the city's various private religious communities.

The leaders of Salt Lake City's more pluralistic religious communities took such responsibilities seriously. By the turn of the twentieth century, they had established schools, libraries, orphans' homes, and other kinds of civic associations for their own congregants in particular, and for the poor, immigrant, and working-class men, women, and children in general.[23] They had also brought hospitals to the territory since the mine and railroad camps surrounding Salt Lake City were full of single men working in high-risk industries plagued by life-threatening accidents and living in the kinds of crowded quarters that bred dreaded infectious diseases. In 1872, the Episcopalians opened St. Mark's Hospital; the Roman Catholic Sisters of the Holy Cross followed with Holy Cross Hospital in 1883. Both hospitals primarily served patients of their own faiths from the surrounding mining and railroad communities. Both St. Mark's and Holy Cross had, in 1894 and 1901, respectively, adopted the then most progressive means of providing competent and efficient day-to-day hospital care for patients by opening their own training schools for nurses.[24]

Mormons and Nursing Care

By the early 1870s, the LDS Church recognized that its traditional ways of caring for the sick were ill-suited to meet the needs of growing communities. The Mormon population in Utah was surging, fueled by both the high birth rates among the settled Mormons and by the immigration of converts from Great Britain, Scandinavia, Germany, and Canada.[25] Moreover, the Mormons emigrating from the eastern urban areas of the United States also brought with them the demand for and knowledge about more expert medical care.[26] In the late 1870s, the church sent a few Mormon women east to receive medical degrees at Philadelphia's Woman's Medical College. They returned to Utah after graduation to practice; to teach midwives, nurses, wives, and mothers; and to set an example of how Mormons might stay true to their faith while also staying abreast of the changing times, changing knowledge, and changing ways of caring for each other and each other's families.[27]

Margaret Curtis Shipp, one of the first Mormon medical graduates of the Woman's Medical College, explicated this new order in her new health magazine, *The Salt Lake Sanitarian*. Linking science, medical practice, nursing, and patient care, Shipp drew clear distinctions between kinds of care offered by different kinds of nursing practitioners. Mothers nursing their sick families at home still had a role. They cared for "ordinary ills," nursed in early and convalescing stages of illness, and made sure their families observed the laws of health that would prevent serious illnesses.[28] But these women were now, in Shipp's words, the "laity." They were informed, but they were not initiated into the complexities of caring for those with dangerous and critical illnesses. This care required skilled, practiced, and knowledgeable nurses. Explicitly acknowledging the importance of trained nurses, Shipp constantly bemoaned the fact that there were often not enough of them in Utah. She approvingly quoted Samuel Gross's 1869 report to the American Medical Association to her laity in the 1888 inaugural edition of the *Sanitarian*. "Were I seriously ill," Gross had written, "and could have but one, the skillful physician or the trained nurse, I would take the nurse every time."[29]

Shipp, other women physicians, and the LDS women's Relief Society had tried to follow the models set by hospitals like those in far-away Philadelphia and nearby Salt Lake City. They opened the Deseret Hospital in 1882, but there ultimately proved to be little community support in the Mormon community for its work. The Relief Society found somewhat more support for its own home nursing and midwifery classes, first established in 1873 and formally organized into the Nurse School in Salt Lake City in 1900.[30] The school claimed three distinct agendas: training midwives, teaching nurses, and instructing young mothers who needed nursing as "a part of every woman's education."[31] Women attended lectures by physicians in contagious diseases, first aid, obstetrics, invalid cooking, public health and hygiene, the care of the sick, and the treatment of common diseases.[32] They then returned to their communities as self-conscious "missionaries" of the new gospel of health, serving families in isolated frontier settlements and individuals in the increasingly urbanized Salt Lake City.[33] Theoretically, the new school would also solve a piece of the problem of the increasing cost of health care for the Mormon middle class. The Relief Society Nurse School promised a free education and an occupational alternative to Mormon women of "modest circumstances" who would, in exchange, provide a set amount of reduced fee or free nursing and midwifery care to their Mormon communities after graduation.[34]

The school never became a popular choice for Mormon women, however. It attracted few lay women interested only in caring for their own families. The demand for midwifery was declining as more and more Mormon women were choosing physicians as birth attendants. And its nurses' work focused only on the care of women and their families after childbirth. This was necessary work, but it remained work that maintained the blurred boundaries between skilled treatments and domestic service.[35] Graduation numbers declined from a high of 32 in 1917 to only 12 by 1921.[36] Relief Society leaders put on a public face of pride in their school's accomplishments, but they voiced private disappointment in the numbers of Mormon women willing to commit to their form of nurses' training.[37]

In fact, more and more Mormon women were training as nurses, but they were choosing to train either in programs established by hospitals throughout the intermountain West, or at St. Mark's in Salt Lake City. These women sought, in particular, medical content, supervised clinical experiences, and experiences that would transform them into formally trained nurses. They sought preparation and instruction that would draw them and their practice away from a traditional focus on home and hearth. They would now be hospital-trained nurses, mediating science and care at the bedside in ways that could not be confused with that of the "laity." The leaders of the Relief Society recognized their claim. In acknowledgment of the new practice of Mormon trained nurses and in response to the demands of the trained nurses themselves, the Relief Society would now formally refer to graduates still in practice as aides and would remind them that, however valuable their care, they were never to give the impression that they were hospital trained.[38]

Mormon student nurses, in fact, had cared for a prominent Mormon dentist, Dr. D. W. Groves, during his 1895 hospitalization at St. Mark's for a heart attack. Groves was one of the increasingly influential members of Salt Lake City's Mormon community who were gradually re-embracing the idea of a hospital as central to the care of isolated and poor individuals, community status, and, increasingly, modern and specialized medical practice. By the turn of the twentieth century, the most modern care meant hospital care, and hospital care meant student nurses' care. With a $50,000 contribution from Groves, the financial support of a now more prosperous Mormon community, and a more financially stable and modern-minded church, the Latter-Day Saints Hospital formally opened in Salt Lake City in 1905. By 1910, it successfully brought formal hospital-based nurses' training to its own Mormon community.

The LDS Hospital Training School for Nurses

When the LDS training school opened, it immediately adopted the then well-known structure of both training and work. Women would trade

three years of their time for scientific knowledge, disciplined representations, and competent and controlled approaches to complicated treatments, medication regimes, aseptic and infection control protocols, and
emergency situations. By the time the LDS Hospital Training School
class of 1919 entered their school, however, the leaders of American
nursing believed a crisis was looming. In their minds, the long hours,
hard work, and distasteful body work seemed to have compromised
nursing's ability to attract the ideal training school candidate. Moreover,
such an ideal nursing candidate now also felt the countervailing pull
of increased opportunities for respectable work in department store
sales or office work that also offered higher salaries and better working conditions.[39]

American nursing leaders were concerned, for they had particular
ideas about the kind of nursing student they wanted and feared they
were not attracting. This student would be female. Indeed, by the time
the LDS class of 1919 graduated, even that last bastion of male
attendance—military nursing—had finally given way to the powerful
combination of paradigmatic femininity and clinical competence.[40] Ideally, the student would also be educated, mature, middle-class, and
white. She would be old enough to have had the life experiences and the
maturity to manage the demands of isolated days and nights with critically ill patients in pain or near death, but she would not be so old as to
be too set in her ways or too tired to physically perform the required
work.

The ideal nurse might also come from a more rural community that
offered fewer educational or social opportunities. If so, then her ambition, dedicated work, discipline, and eagerness to learn the lessons of
character as well as clinical training would open worlds to her that had
previously seemed unattainable. She could travel, she could achieve financial independence, and she could claim respected and respectable
work. A woman wanting to nurse might also come from a working-class
background. But unlike most other working-class women, a woman
who would nurse would come from financially secure working-class
households that did not need her unpaid labor or her immediate wages
during the three years of training.[41] She had to have accumulated sufficient capital to pay for uniforms, books, and equipment such as syringes
and scissors that she had to bring with her to her chosen school. She

came, that is, from upper-working-class families ready to launch their sons and daughters into the bottom tiers of the new middle class.[42]

For all of organized nursing's concern, however, the members of the LDS Hospital Training School Class of 1919 did seem to represent what American nursing leaders wanted. All were white women. These graduates were also precisely the right age. The oldest member of the class, Maria Johnson, graduated at thirty-one; the youngest, Pearl Blackburn, graduated at twenty-two. Most women, however, were between twenty-three and twenty-four when they graduated. Most of the 1919 graduates were also native born, with long roots in the United States on one or both sides of their families. Of these graduates, 69 percent had two native-born parents; 23 percent had one parent born abroad in France, Sweden, and Ireland respectively; and only Clara Wall was the child of two immigrant parents. Most graduates (69 percent) were born in Utah; others (31 percent) were born in Mormon communities in Nevada, Wyoming, and Idaho. Some 15 percent of the class of 1919 were born in the urban centers of Salt Lake City and Provo. Most others, however, were born in the small towns that settled the Wasatch Front moving south from Salt Lake City. A few came from the small towns and isolated settlements scattered throughout the state and the intermountain region (Table 4.1).

The graduates of the class of 1919 were born into large Mormon families. They averaged eleven living siblings each: two graduates had fourteen living siblings; three claimed the low of only seven. Some of these graduates' families may have been poor in material resources but not necessarily in social status. Almost half of the graduates of the class of 1919 for whom data are available (35% of the total class) came from families only one generation removed from the practice of polygamy. Their grandparents had the plural marriages that had traditionally been the prerogative of the Mormon social elite. Plural marriage was essential to men's aspirations to influential church careers, and it increased the likelihood that women would be appointed to leadership positions with the Relief Society.[43]

Moreover, plural marriage increased the likelihood that these particular graduates of the class of 1919 saw their grandmothers making substantive contributions to their families' economic and social prosperity. Plural wives often worked, either selling farm products in the market or in salaried positions both to help support their extended families and, at

TABLE 4.1 Graduates of the Latter-Day Saints Hospital Training School, class of 1919

	Year of birth	Place of birth	No. living siblings	Location of entry into training school	Year married	Age at marriage (years)	No. of children
A. Roberts[a]	1896	Polk, MO	7	Kemmerer, WY	1923	27	1
B. Ashby[a]	1897	Summitt, UT	8	Bountiful, UT	1920	23	5
V. Caldwell	N/A	N/A	N/A	St. Johns, UT			0
L. Bassett[a,b]	1897	White Plains, NV	9	American Fork, UT	1924	27	2
S. Yancy[a,c]	1897	Bancock, ID	14	Blackfoot, ID	1917	20	7
L. Peck	1894	Box Elder, UT	7	Cove, OR	1921	27	2
M. Thatcher	1893	Unita, WY	8	Blackfoot, ID	1918	25	N/A
M. Sandberg[a]	N/A	St. George, UT	8	St. George, UT	N/A	N/A	4
L. Tooth	1896	Sanpete, UT	11	Mante, UT	1924	28	2
R. Kerr	N/A	N/A	N/A	Provo, UT	N/A	N/A	1
M. Johnson	1888	Springville, UT	8	Springville, UT			0
N. Armitstead[d]	1893	Provo, UT	11	Provo, UT	1918	25	2
R. Farnsworth	1897	N/A	12	Provo, UT	1923	26	N/A
F. Hansen[a]	N/A	N/A	N/A	Salt Lake City			N/A
P. Blackburn	1898	Loa, UT	14	Loa, UT	1924	26	N/A
C. Wall	1893	Salt Lake City	N/A	Lyman, WY	N/A	N/A	0
I. Knowlton[d]	1893	N/A	7	Salt Lake City	1922	29	1

SOURCE: The History of the LDS Hospital School of Nursing, 1905–1955 and, when available, the Ancestral File Notes, Family History Library, Church of Jesus Christ of Latter-day Saints, Salt Lake City, Utah (also available at www.familysearch.org/eng/default.asp).

[a]Reported that she never worked for wages.
[b]Died in 1929 of tuberculosis.
[c]Died in childbirth (year unknown).
[d]Reported that she never nursed for wages.
N/A = not available.

times, to allow some sister-wives to pursue professional careers. But by the early 1900s it was equally likely that these graduates saw their mothers reclaiming (in wish, if not in fact) more conventionally domestic roles as wives and mothers as the LDS church moved closer to mainstream American norms.

The women in the LDS Training School class of 1919 graduated from a school that had begun, as did most training schools, as a small endeavor and then grew in both numbers of students and in the length of training as the number of hospital beds and procedures performed increased. Like other such institutions, the LDS Hospital needed more and more student nurse staffing. By 1914, the LDS Training School was graduating, on average, sixteen to twenty women each year. But the demand continued to increase, and its wards and operating rooms easily absorbed the work of the thirty-five students who graduated in the class of 1917 and the twenty-nine graduates of the class of 1920. But the classes of 1918, 1919, and 1920 also found themselves fighting an unexpected and deadly 1918 flu pandemic. The pandemic hit Utah first in Salt Lake City and then moved relentlessly south along the highway that linked the more settled Wasatch Front.[44] The graduates of the LDS Training School class of 1919 remained curiously silent about their work during the pandemic. The class of 1918, however, mourned the deaths of two fellow students who were infected with the virus when caring for these patients.[45]

These women also graduated from a training school that was the jewel in the crown of a slowly growing number of Mormon-run hospitals and training schools throughout Utah.[46] It had the most beds, the most money, and the most prestige. As significantly, its training school met the still-voluntary criteria for excellence in education and practice that had been established by the American Nurses Association and the National League for Nursing Education, the two most important national nursing associations. The hospital had a sufficient number of beds to provide varied clinical experiences. The training school curriculum provided lectures in substantive areas of nursing practice, and its graduates met certain standards that involved prior educational experiences, character screening, and professional competency.

All student nurses worked hard. Their clinical work included the preparation of individualized diabetic meals that contained precisely measured amounts of fat, carbohydrates, and proteins; treating patients with lead poisoning (the most common reason for hospitalization among miners) with draughts of sodium chloride mixed in a tincture of chloride iron; and drawing and monitoring the temperature of the tepid baths needed by those with typhoid fever contacted in the overcrowded settlements of the railroad communities. Students also replaced continuous hot packs every three hours on the chests of patients with pneumonia and mixed and applied the then-ubiquitous mustard and flaxseed poultices prescribed for almost every other condition. The more talented students assisted surgeons in the operating rooms, and the most talented ones gained supervisory experience as head nurses and instructors of novice students on patient wards.[47]

Most of the students' days, however, involved housecleaning, laundry, and other chores that were at once mundane and yet, in their contribution to the hygiene, cleanliness, and comfort of the ward environment, absolutely critical to the recovery of ill patients. Much of the work demanded by the LDS Hospital Training School, as was that of so many training schools across the country, was "just plain hard labor." Nor was it work that even the most sanguine graduate might describe as an uplifting experience. Rhea Kerr, one graduate of the class of 1919, who herself became a superintendent of nurses at an LDS hospital in Idaho Falls, Idaho, in 1923, took pride in her singular accomplishment. She claimed she went through her entire training without ever emptying a bed pan. Graduates felt little need to romanticize or sentimentalize their work. "Well," remembered Lettie Sorenson Mickelson, a graduate of the class of 1909, "we managed."[48]

Race, relative resources, and the wish to travel to Salt Lake City to train as nurses seemed to be the only commonalities among the graduates of the class of 1919. Indeed, the graduates knew themselves to be a socially, geographically, and financially diverse group. They tried to mitigate at least the more egregious markings of these kinds of disparities. They had watched at other graduations as the "girls from well-to-do families got so many flowers that they could not carry them off stage." Others, they noted, "received small nosegays, some none at all." At their own graduation ceremony, they decided to do away with the practice of carrying flowers. In their minds, "it just wasn't fair."[49]

Still, we know little about why the graduates of the class of 1919 wanted to become nurses.[50] Some of their colleagues in other LDS

Training School classes did, however, write about their recollected reasons for choosing nursing. These reasons, not surprisingly, were not quite as altruistic as those most probably penned in the obligatory admission applications. But their recollections do show the strong support of both their families and their communities of faith and friends—support that at once reflected traditional roles and authority relationships and that acknowledged the possibility of their practice in more contemporary and less conventional arenas. Frieda Jensen Stelter's mother had heard about the "new" training school at her Relief Society meeting and believed it to be a good place for her daughter. Others, such as Clara Duncombe Beach, received encouragement from their community's physicians. As Margaret Ingersol remembered, one such physician specifically told her to enroll in the LDS Hospital Training School. He believed it an alternative to "wasting her time in a small town." Ingersol did, and after graduation she enlisted in the Army Nurse Corps when the United States entered World War I. She retired from the army as a colonel.[51]

Still other remembrances suggest that LDS graduates, however strong their religious convictions and altruistic desires, also kept one eye firmly focused on the social realities. Their reasons were quite pragmatic. Both Esther Wixon Johnson and Willmerth Skinner Elton Bently were widows responsible for the support of their children. Their parents and their communities helped care for their children while they were in training. Still others showed a particular joining of religion, realism, and personal ambition. Mae Jenson Thomson, for example, thought ahead to a future in which she might need to support herself and chose the LDS Nurses Training School because she could not afford college.[52]

Indeed, for many of the LDS Training School graduates, a nursing diploma did become the stepping-stone to a collegiate degree. Nursing work allowed such women to eventually accumulate the necessary social and financial resources that turned a collegiate education into a dream deferred, not a dream denied. At the University of Utah, where most of the LDS Training School graduates matriculated, nursing school graduates received academic credits for training school coursework, and these credits significantly shortened the time needed to pursue degrees in public health nursing, administration, or education. In all, 18 percent of the graduates of the class of 1919 had earned a collegiate degree by the time they responded to their 1955 alumnae association survey. This was quite a significant accomplishment: in 1955 only 10.4 percent of all nurses nationally had earned a baccalaureate degree; only 7.8 percent of all white women nationally could claim such an achievement.[53]

Charlotte Dancy, the superintendent of nurses at the LDS Hospital and the head of its Training School during the three years the class of 1919 spent at the hospital, serves as one strong example of how nursing might open new roles for Mormon women in ways that still valued traditional commitments. Dancy, the fourth of ten children born into a socially prominent North Carolina family, had graduated from Baltimore's prestigious Johns Hopkins Hospital School of Nursing. She had been quickly hired in 1902 by the newly formed Newark, New Jersey, Visiting Nurse Association (VNA) as its first trained nurse. Dancy, like other visiting nurses, provided the physical care that its immigrant and working-class patients needed, but also, and just as importantly, she used her personality and her presence as a tool to inspire them, their families, and their friends to adopt more modern, healthier, and more American habits and customs.

As with all visiting nurses, what Dancy did and who she was remained intricately connected. She moved in the wider world as the quintessential role model of informed, educated, and single womanhood. Dancy came to the LDS Training School for Nurses after she converted to the Mormon faith and emigrated to Utah. The choice to remain unmarried in a church that so privileged marriage and motherhood had serious social repercussions, but such a choice could be redeemed by a life devoted to service. Dancy led the school until 1922, when she joined the faculty of the new Utah State University, where she remained a role model. She became dean of women at USU in 1925 and served until 1930, also teaching classes in home health, nursing, anatomy, and physiology.[54]

Under Dancy's watchful eyes, the graduates of the class of 1919 managed a social life during their training that could, if these students so chose, set the stage for marriage and motherhood. Indeed, the entry of the United States into World War I in 1917 dramatically highlighted the graduates' romantic relationships. Sylvia Yancy, for example, immediately married Jared Anderson in 1917 at the beginning of her second year in training, just before he went overseas with the army. Yancy had

Dancy's permission.[55] Neola Armitstead, who married Freeman Gross in 1918, her third year of training, also presumably had permission. But Margaret Thatcher either could not or would not get such permission. Undeterred, she married James Shaw in 1918. Thatcher soon became pregnant, which not surprisingly "caused much consternation among her class friends." The penalty would have been an immediate dismissal. But Thatcher, like Yancy and Armitstead, graduated with her class. Dancy never discovered either the marriage or the pregnancy.[56]

It is possible, as historian Kathryn McPherson has argued, that Dancy did know but deliberately turned a blind eye to the situation.[57] Second-year nursing students like Yancey already represented an enormous investment in time and teaching. Moreover, third-year students like Thatcher were precisely at the point in their training where such an investment had begun to yield dividends of increasingly skilled, resourceful, and independent patient care. Nursing students certainly appreciated this fact. There were no conventional strikes that labor historians frequently look to for evidence of workplace activism, but the LDS Hospital Training School students fully knew the power of collective action in furthering what they believed to be their own self-interest. Vilate Caldwell, herself a graduate of the class of 1919 and Dancy's successor as the superintendent of the LDS training school, learned how they might do so. Caldwell had warned her nursing students that they would lose the privilege of wearing their nurses' cap if they chose to bob their hair; she saw the increasingly fashionable idea of cutting one's long hair short as an act of social rebellion. The students "decided to ignore the threat" and did cut their hair. When confronted, they surrendered their caps—and their uniforms as well. Caldwell relented in the face of this informal work stoppage, and the following week, the class historian noted gleefully, all the nursing instructors bobbed their own hair.[58]

Caldwell remained single and chose, like her classmate Maria Johnson, "a purely professional career."[59] One other classmate, Clara Wall, also chose a lifelong career as a nurse. Wall, however, came from a different background than Caldwell and Johnson and had a different kind of career. Wall's father and mother were Mormon immigrants from Sweden and Denmark. She entered training at the LDS Hospital in 1916 and remained employed there after graduation. Wall served at first as a general duty nurse, caring for patients and supervising the students who still performed most of the hospital's nursing care. In 1923 Wall was promoted to the position of night nursing supervisor. She was one of the most experienced clinicians in the hospital, making rounds to organize, oversee, and support the work of younger nursing staff, students, and quite often medical interns from midnight to seven in the morning. By 1939, Wall had earned better hours and the position of evening nursing supervisor, a position she held for more than fifteen years. Like Caldwell and Johnson, Wall was a faithful church member, but her professional ambitions were tied more tightly to both the LDS Hospital and to the needs of her family. Her proudest accomplishment, she wrote her class-mates in 1954, was that her paid work gave her brother and two nephews the financial freedom to serve as evangelizing missionaries for the Mormon Church in the United States and abroad.[60] Wall worked at the LDS Hospital until her death in 1964.

Most (79%) of the graduates of the class of 1919 married, however. The LDS Hospital Nurses' Alumnae Association despaired that such married graduates rarely participated in the initiatives and the events of their organization.[61] But married graduates had, by and large, moved on to another way of life and were traveling along different life paths.

The Life Paths of Married Graduates, Class of 1919

As both contemporaries and historians have long recognized, most married nurses followed a fairly typical life-cycle work path. They worked before they married. They then left the workforce while raising their children and sometimes returned when their children left home. May Ayres Burgess's 1928 data on workforce participation showed employment rates falling precipitously from a high of 91 percent three years after graduation to 20 percent ten years after graduation before bottoming at 5 percent twenty years after graduation when presumably forty-something nurses would be deeply involved with their families. Workforce participation rates plateaued for a time, then began slowly rising. Nine percent of nurses worked twenty-five years after their graduation, and as many as 25 percent had returned to work forty years after their training school graduations.[62]

The married graduates of the class of 1919 followed this aggregate life-cycle trend of work and marriage, dropping out of the wage labor market while raising children and then sometimes returning to paid employment when their children left home. But such patterns mask significant trends in their lives after training.[63] On average, the married graduates of the class of 1919 for whom substantive data are available (eleven of fourteen) worked for three years after graduation. They married at twenty-six, and, although they themselves had come from large families, the married 1919 graduates had only, on average, two children (Table 4.1). In all, the 1919 LDS Training School graduates married much later and had significantly fewer children than Mormon women peers in particular, and American women in general. In one generation, LDS nursing women from the class of 1919 had achieved marriage and fertility patterns that mirrored that of mainstream, middle-class America rather than that of their Mormon peers, who still married younger and had substantially higher birthrates (Table 4.1).[64]

Of course, prolonged courtships, older ages at marriage, and fewer children have long been, as historians and demographers have pointed out, very effective strategies for families aspiring to and maintaining middle-class status.[65] Such strategies gave individuals the time necessary to acquire an education that promised the successful occupational positions that would increase one's material resources and standard of living. An eight-year courtship, for example, allowed Samuel Lindsay time to establish a business with his brother and to build a home for his fiancée, Alice Powell. Powell was one of the Mormon women who wanted to be a nurse prior to the establishment of the LDS Hospital Training School but did not share the Relief Society vision of home nurses training; she received her hospital-based nursing education at Michigan's Battle Creek Sanatorium. During her eight-year courtship, Powell worked as an assistant nursing supervisor at the then newly opened LDS Hospital and took courses in public health nursing at the University of Utah. This proved fortunate, for Lindsay died suddenly of pneumonia in 1932, and Powell had to return to work to support her young family. She worked first as a visiting nurse, often, during the depths of the Great Depression, exchanging her services for produce to feed her children. Powell soon secured a school nursing position with the Salt Lake County Public Health Department. School nursing complemented rather than competed with her family commitments. This position, she remembered, "enabled me to be home most of the time when the children were there."[66]

Still, as Powell well knew, the place of lower-middle- and middle-class Americans just above the early twentieth-century line between comfort and poverty was often quite tenuous. Marriage, in fact, provided few guarantees of a life of leisure or even economic security. When women looked around their communities, they saw well over half of their married sisters with children working full-time, some 20 percent for wages (as reported in official census statistics), but an additional (and never officially counted) 30 percent working for free in their families' small businesses or on their farms.[67] Moreover, the loss of a salaried position, a failure in a business enterprise, an untimely death, or the dissolution of a marriage could as easily send a family back down the social ladder.[68] Indeed, the pragmatism of the graduates of the class of 1919 had a basis in the realities of their own and their community's lives. Some had lost parents; others experienced the effects of divorce.

As economists have long pointed out, when families have skilled workers in reserve and ready to re-enter the labor market when social and economic hardship strikes, they can often stabilize their finances and maintain their standards of living. Hence, the graduates' pragmatism had its own rewards. One 1919 graduate, Arline Peck, married Paul Ross in 1921. Peck was twenty-seven when she married, and she continued working as a visiting nurse for the Metropolitan Life Insurance Company while her husband completed his education and traveled on missions for the LDS Church. Peck's marriage ultimately crumbled. She returned to work at an outpatient clinic near a mining site to support herself and her two sons.

Bonds forged in training also helped. When Roxana Farnsworth's husband died in 1935, few patients could afford the private duty nursing care she thought she might provide to support herself and her three young children. However, her classmate Maria Johnson, now director of nursing at the LDS Hospital, stepped in and appointed her to a secure, stable, and reasonably well-paid position on the hospital's general duty staff.[69] Whatever happened, all the graduates of the class of 1919 who wanted to could get a job as a nurse.

But nursing represented more than just a pragmatic economic strategy. It also allowed some women the possibility of imagining themselves in new kinds of roles and relationships that provided alternatives to traditional paths. A later LDS training school graduate, Violet Larsson, may have given voice to a more common experience: she imagined a lifelong nursing career as a single woman and struggled to reconcile that dream with an equally powerful one about marriage. Larsson, it seems, knew the handsome Joseph Olpin from their high school days. But when he reappeared at the LDS training school doors after missionary and military service, Larsson decided to avoid him. As her daughter remembered, Larsson had "strong feelings" for Olpin, but she was afraid these feelings "would interfere with the life career she had chosen." Olpin persisted in his attention, and Larsson prayed and sought a blessing from her bishop to help her decide between career or marriage. Larsson did decide to marry Olpin immediately after her graduation in 1921. Together, they built a successful mortuary and ambulance business. Larsson eventually did what she called "some active nursing." Every other month she filled in for a vacationing nurse at the nearby American Fork Hospital, some twenty miles south of Salt Lake City. And with enormous pride, she saw two of her daughters graduate from the Brigham Young University School of Nursing.[70]

The point of Larsson's story lies less in her choice of marriage and more in her choice of marriage as one of several salient options. It is also significant that Larsson worked both before and after her marriage and children, and that her work included both unpaid labor within her family's ambulance service and part-time paid labor outside. Part-time and intermittent patterns of wage labor figure prominently in the life stories of nursing school graduates. In Utah, the American Fork Hospital, in particular, depended on the occasional work of married nurses with families when it unexpectedly had too many patients for its general duty nursing staff. Alice Smith Aylett, a 1926 graduate of Salt Lake City's Holy Cross Hospital Training School, remembered, "When my youngest was a baby . . . I helped the night nurse when she had maternity patients in the early hours." Aylett's community had yet to receive telephone service. When her assistance was needed, she said, "the sheriff would come and get me."[71] Life stories from the LDS Hospital class of 1919 also suggest such part-time and intermittent employment patterns that emerged hand in hand with the growing hospital system throughout early twentieth-century Utah. Two 1919 graduates sometimes worked in physicians' offices, and others reported that they "did some nursing."

Lucy Tooth, in particular, worked on and off "for years as the mainstay of the Saline Valley Hospital."[72]

Given such a range of options, it seems surprising that 57 percent of the married graduates of the class of 1919 never in their lifetimes worked in salaried nursing positions. For example, Irene Knowlton, the class "fashion plate," took a sales position in the infants department of the Paris Department Store immediately after her graduation. There, her classmates noted, "she was in her glory advising expectant, and indeed all, mothers." Knowlton eventually married three years after graduation and raised one son. Most of the other married graduates who never worked in a salaried nursing position, however, never worked outside the home at all. Marilla Sandberg Fitzgerald, otherwise known as "Miss Sunshine," returned to her hometown of St. George, Utah, married, and raised four sons. She and four other of her classmates concentrated, in the words of Neola Armistead, on "only nursing their families."[73] Most of these graduates married soon after graduation and, one assumes, met their future husbands either before or during their training school experience. Two 1919 graduates died when still quite young. Leah Bassett's death from tuberculosis reflected the ever-present dangers still confronting early twentieth-century nurses. Sylvia Yancy's death in childbirth reflected another danger that confronted early twentieth-century women (Table 4.1).

Certainly, some women who entered nurses training quickly discovered that they loathed the hard work, the relentless demands, the rigid hierarchy, and the strict discipline that characterized early twentieth-century nurses training. But many of these women would have left or would have been asked to leave the LDS training school almost as soon as they arrived. "Even Florence Nightingale," Ruth Partridge decided when reflecting on her own early twentieth-century nurses training "would have been expelled from any up-to-date hospital." No nursing supervisor, she wrote, would have tolerated her "prowling around at night with a lamp, breaking up routines, and by-passing the authority of her superiors." Although Partridge never names her hospital or training school, she does give one reason why she, and perhaps some others, stayed. "It's just stubbornness. . . . Your folks or some friend who is a nurse says you can't stick it out, and you stick it out just to show them."[74]

Partridge stuck it out. And then she, in her description, collapsed into the arms of her fiancé on her graduation day and never nursed a day in her life thereafter.

The rhetoric, of course, was also that nursing school might prepare one to be a better wife and mother. It would take a young woman with some aptitude and use hospital routines and expectations to teach her how to manage a house, promote healthy and moral lifestyles among her children, and, when necessary, care for sick kin. Yet the graduates of the LDS Training School never spoke to this rhetoric when reflecting on their training school experiences. Perhaps it seemed so understood that it needed no explication, and certainly an alumnae survey might be an unlikely place to boast about unpaid domestic housework and care work with colleagues claiming significant accomplishments in the paid labor market. But married Mormon nurses who never worked for wages took enormous pride in their community work and in the services they provided. For example, Amelia Latta, an 1895 graduate of St. Luke's Training School in Denver, Colorado, never worked after her marriage and her move to Provo, Utah. But "because she was a trained nurse," her biographer remembered, "people of the entire community called on [her] in time of sickness. If a child had the measles, if a man had an accident, or if a woman needed help in the days after childbirth, the call was to 'go for Sister Latta.'"[75] Similarly, Lettie Sorenson Mickelson, a 1909 LDS Training School graduate who had married and moved to Hollywood in 1917, continued nursing, providing private duty care both in homes and hospitals. And, she added proudly, "I never charged anything for my services."[76]

A New Social Space for Nurses

As many historians have pointed out, early twentieth-century American women created a social space in which largely white, single women from a variety of class backgrounds increasingly experimented with different kinds of paid work options, new forms of cooperative relationships, freedom from familial supervision, the pleasures of sexuality, and the diverse challenges that accompanied their quest, however temporary, for economic independence.[77] In many ways, the LDS Hospital Training School for Nurses created this same kind of space for a particular group of Mormon women who wanted to experience the promise of individual self-fulfillment *and* remain faithful to their church's pro-marriage, pro-family, and pronatalist teachings. Their three-year training school experience gave them specialized skills in care work, a feel for their own power and expertise when defending personal interests, and just as importantly, time away from home to experiment with the implications of and, for some, to postpone or even change life choices.

The class of 1919, in fact, graduated and began their paid work lives at precisely the same age, twenty-two, that their Mormon sisters were already married and considering motherhood. They looked, not to a job, but to a particular career in service—a career that muted dramatic shifts in self-perception as they moved between their wage work, housework, and care work, and a career that reinterpreted Mormon women's traditional roles in health and healing even as their church moved to increasingly limit their religious roles and their formal organizational authority. Moreover, even if the LDS Church might not actively encourage the personal ambitions of married women outside their homes and families, it also placed few roadblocks in the life paths chosen by the LDS Training School graduates.

Certainly, these particular Mormon women were never entirely free of the demands of their family's domestic economy. But if not entirely free, such women were not entirely trapped either. They had salient opportunities and choices within their families' social place, and their paid and unpaid work (sometimes alone, sometimes in partnership with husbands) made significant contributions to its rising social location. These women shared their church's position on the value of their roles as women, wives, and mothers, but they also worked to meet their own needs as well as those of their family. In the end, they participated in the construction of a rather fluid domestic space that responded fairly well to the complicated and often quite personal negotiations among a religion's dictates, an individual's desires, a child's needs, the value of a husband's work, and the unpredictability of certain economic and social realities both at particular moments and over the course of a lifetime. The choice of nursing work, then, was an effective strategy for some Mormon women who sought to reconcile conflicting desires, demands, and expectations in their personal and professional lives.

This new social space had significant problems. The promise of nursing work did not always match reality as married nurses in the wage labor market often confronted poor working conditions both in private duty and in hospitals. Moreover, the constant movement of married nurses in and out of, as well as between, various occupational positions within the wage labor market prevented a sustained critique of working conditions that might have led to change. Single nurses without families of their own to turn to in cases of their own illnesses or accidents remained extraordinarily vulnerable when unable to work and support themselves financially.

This social space remained one largely accessible only to married white women. Many married African American nurses, sometimes by choice but more often by racial practices that sharply curtailed the employment options and opportunities of African American men, had to continue to work in paid employment to help support themselves and their families. The Freedmen's Hospital nursing alumnae gathered the life stories of the graduates of the school's first fifty years in preparation for a centennial celebration in 1984, much in the same way the LDS graduates did for 1955 celebration.[78] Only a small number of its early graduates remained alive. But among those who did contribute, stories emerged of an assumption almost taken for granted that its African American nursing graduates would continue to work after marriage. Irene Scott Williams, a 1916 graduate, wrote of a chronology of positions she held within and outside nursing while married and raising her two children. She worked as a visiting nurse with the Metropolitan Life Insurance Company in Atlanta and as a supervisor of a nursery school in Detroit before she retired in 1957 from the Detroit Board of Education. She still had time to attend Wayne State University, Kalamazoo State Teachers College, and the University of Michigan, taking courses in psychology, sociology, and early childhood education and development.[79] Only Aileen Cole Stewart, a 1917 graduate, alluded to the difficulties of maintaining these kinds of commitments. "By careful planning of my time and use of my resources and income, I did not have any difficulty managing my nursing career and raising a family."[80] She pointed with pride to the achievements of her daughter, Jean Theresa Stewart, an accomplished poet and author.[81]

But the construction of this kind of social space did work for one group of nurses. For all their differences, this particular group shared ambition and a set of values that remained faithful to more conservative notions of individualism and self-reliance and to more traditional ideas about women and about how women might weigh personal aspirations against the equally compelling needs of their families. This group—a group that certainly included Mormon nurses but that also included many others—might have chafed at the public's seeming subordination of their nursing work to that of physician and hospitals. But their attention to their nursing work was only a piece of a broader calculus about the significance of their work within their families and their communities as well as within their chosen profession. To them, nursing was not only about the work but also about the meaning of the work. To them, nursing meant choices and opportunities they would not otherwise have had. To them, nursing held the promise of individual self-fulfillment *and* faithfulness to the needs of their families.

CHAPTER 5

Race, Place, and Professional Identity

O N OCTOBER 28, 1929, Jane Van de Vrede, the executive secretary of the Georgia State Nurses Association, rose to address her regional colleagues at the inaugural meeting of the Southern Division of the American Nurses Association.[1] The Southern Division, she reminded them, would follow in the footsteps of those created by Northeastern nurses in 1919, Northwestern nurses in 1921, Mid-Atlantic nurses in 1925, and Midwestern nurses in 1927. It would promote the promise and the possibilities of nursing in the region, provide a site for the interchange of ideas, and bring nurses in the South into "closer fellowship." More to the point, she noted, the Southern Division's meetings of white nurses from Alabama, Arkansas, Florida, Georgia, Kentucky, Louisiana, Mississippi, North Carolina, Oklahoma, South Carolina, Tennessee, Texas, Virginia, and West Virginia would provide a forum to discuss issues pertinent only to the region—issues that would not and should not make the floor of national nursing conventions.

Certainly, Van de Vrede continued, there were many such issues that contributed to what she described as the "particularity of the south." The region's growing urban areas did have some larger hospitals, with the requisite numbers of beds and clinical services that provided the necessary content and formative experiences that national nursing leaders believed essential to the training of nurses. But most hospitals in the South tended to be small, private, and specialized. Many with formal nurses training schools had fewer than twenty-five beds and even fewer patients on any given day. Van de Vrede did not need to remind her audience how this regional reality played out on a national stage. By 1929, American nursing leadership stood adamantly opposed to training schools in small hospitals with limited clinical and educational opportunities.[2] They constantly criticized the role these small schools played in creating what they explicitly called a "two-class nursing system" of well-trained and poorly trained women, and they dreaded the prospect that it might create opportunities for completely untrained women "passing" as more formally trained nurses.[3]

The socially resonant references to a "two-class system" and the racially freighted language of "passing" reflected American nursing leadership's deeply held fears that nursing's carefully constructed identity could too easily disintegrate into class- and race-based stereotypes. This seemed especially problematic in the American south. As Van de Vrede pointed out to her colleagues, the idea of nursing that had been born in the exploits of Florence Nightingale and that had come of age in the needs of patients in hospitals still "challenged the woman of culture" in the South.[4] Middle- and upper-class white and African American southern women seeking opportunities to make meaningful contributions to their kin and communities most often chose church and club work; they only rarely chose opportunities to nurse (for money) those with whom they claimed no blood or community ties. The more routine and tedious work of the day-to-day nursing of strangers—most of nursing's work—was still done by working-class white servants and by African Americans, who still bore the burden of roles associated with slavery.[5]

The idea, the identity, and the practice of a formally trained nurse had, in many ways, a national scope. As in the North and the West, the idea of a trained nurse promised southern women the opportunity to engage with valued and valuable medical knowledge. Their training school experience promised the same trial by fire that forged a strong sense of their power, their ability, and their value. And they learned similar practices and procedures needed to care for the sick in homes and hospitals. This chapter, however, moves south to Georgia, and to Atlanta in particular—to Van de Vrede's beloved "New South" city in the heart of one of the strongest bastions of Jim Crow in the United States. Here the idea, the identity, and the practices of trained nurses played themselves out in a context riven with deeply held assumptions and openly expressed tensions about how class and race determined one's role in the care of the sick.

This chapter examines the aspirations, the educational opportunities, and the work experiences of both white and African American nurses in Georgia in the first half of the twentieth century. It considers the complicated intersections of class, race, and nursing identities as these nurses worked simultaneously side by side and in completely separate worlds. It explores how the idea and the identity of trained nurses were not just willed and constructed—but also contested. Georgia's white and African American nurses lived and worked in a place quite unlike those of cosmopolitan New York or Mormon Utah. But their experiences are as instructive. They suggest that both the idea and the identity of trained nurses depended on women willing to do the work of nursing—on women willing to trade their work for meaningful, respected, and authoritative medical knowledge. But they also depended on powerful social support for the women who would do such work. White and African American women in Georgia found that lacking. This was especially apparent in its capital, Atlanta.

Nursing in the "New South City"

Atlanta, like other growing, industrializing, and commercializing southern cities, saw itself as all that was new and modern and progressive in the early twentieth-century South. With an official seal of a phoenix rising from the ashes of Civil War destruction, and under the tutelage of Henry Grady, the editor of the *Atlanta Constitution* and one of the city's biggest boosters, the "Atlanta spirit" promised a sustained commitment to urban growth, opportunity, and an abiding faith that the city could meet all challenges in its quest to be the premier "New South City." Its International Cotton Exposition of 1881, modeled on Philadelphia's Centennial Fair of 1876, drew the attention of northern textile manufacturers to the region's cotton belt, on the one hand, and to the city's extensive railroad connections to northern and midwestern markets on the other. Its 1895 Cotton States and International Exposition highlighted what the city believed to be its progressive stance on race relations. Booker T. Washington, the nationally known proponent of African American economic initiative, impressed and reassured a predominately white audience in a speech that would later become known as the "Atlanta Compromise."[6] Washington, hoping to reconcile the interests of all Americans, painted a picture of African American men and women seeking only economic self-sufficiency and temporarily setting aside political aspirations despite an increasingly and more rigidly segregated society. Soon after Washington's speech, the U.S. Supreme Court's decision in *Plessy vs. Ferguson* affirmed "separate but equal" as national public policy.[7]

There was a dark side to this "New South City." The Atlanta Race Riot of 1906 laid bare the extent to which the city's ideology depended upon its willingness to resort to violence to enforce white supremacy.[8] Northern African American reformers shunned the city. For Algernon Jackson, the chair of the department of Public Health and Hygiene at Howard University in Washington, D.C., Atlanta was a place "in the middle of hell."[9] The city deliberately underfunded its educational and public health care systems lest tax dollars support African American institutions. The influx of working-class white women to its mills and offices stoked racial fears about how to protect southern white womanhood.[10] Tuberculosis was rampant among poor men, women, and children of all races. For a city claiming to be a model of southern progressivism, there was little sustained attention to the needs of its most destitute, vulnerable, and, invariably, its sickest citizens.[11]

White reformers, admiring the success of northern cities in attending to the needs of its sick poor and hoping to model their institutions, could point to Grady Memorial Hospital, opened in 1892 and named in honor of Henry Grady, who had died in 1889. Like all urban hospitals throughout the nation, Grady, as it was commonly called, stood as the city's testament to bringing the best in medical treatment and nursing care to its poor. Given strict segregation laws and customs, it did so in carefully constructed and physically separate sections for white and African American patients. White patients, as the outspoken African American physician Henry Butler noted, stayed in an architecturally impressive and spacious brick building. But, he continued, a city that promoted itself as full of "push, pluck, and Christian progress" relegated its African American patients to a small, overcrowded wooden annex next to the institution's kitchen.[12]

White Nurses at Grady

The nurses' training school came to Grady in much the same way it came to other American hospitals. The Grady Memorial Hospital Aid Association had formed at the hospital's opening as a volunteer committee of white and wealthy women committed to visiting the wards, encouraging individual patients, and raising money for the books, newspapers, flowers, and other "delicacies" that the city would not subsidize.[13] But unlike women in other such associations throughout the country, the white women of the Aid Association immediately confronted the color line that they decided not to cross. A brief experiment bringing songs to the African American wards on Sundays stopped with the decision to confine their activities to the white wards and with vague notions of inviting African American women to assume such responsibilities on the African American wards.[14]

The Grady Aid Association, like others, also assumed responsibility for organizing nursing care. They had visited the Roosevelt Hospital in New York City and quickly decided that Roosevelt's "neatness and elegance" was due in large part to the nurses in its training school.[15] Again they confronted the color line that they did not want to cross. A training school for white women would open fairly quickly, but the nursing care of African American patients remained problematic. The Aid Association considered the possibility of asking Spelman Seminary, a private school for African American women established by the Woman's American Baptist Home Mission and supported by John D. Rockefeller, to send women in its nurses training program to the Grady Hospital. Spelman had been the first nursing program in Georgia for any woman of any background, and the institution had its own small hospital. But Grady's Board of Trustees tersely dismissed the idea as "impractical."[16]

The Grady Memorial Hospital Training School for Nurses, opened to white students in 1898, had a stumbling start. The medical staff warned the Aid Association that the training school would never attract the "best class" of nurses unless they were moved from their "uncomfortable" rooms on the hospital's third floor into a residence of their own. In the North, separate nurses' homes were quickly becoming a symbol of a hospital's commitment to provide social and sexual protection to women whose education and work challenged conventional understandings of proper roles and responsibilities. The self-styled "old fashioned" and founding members of the Grady Aid Association were willing to spend money on such a nurses' home, but they remained locked for years in a battle with newer and younger members less interested in nursing and more committed to raising money for a new children's ward.[17]

The day-to-day problems were significant. Some were connected to the conflation of gender, race, and acceptable practices in the South. The white female nursing students continuously complained about unseemly contact with male African American patients when they were required to bathe them, even though an ad hoc committee of hospital trustees and physicians assured them that their survey of other southern hospitals showed that this was an accepted practice and not a breach of the color line.[18] Other problems were more common to schools across the country. Nursing superintendents and supervisors came and went; the visiting families of the white students constantly upset hospital routines; and rumors circulated that some nurses broke with propriety and spent evenings with former patients at unseemly "places of amusement."[19]

Annie Bess Feebeck, a 1909 Grady Hospital Training School graduate, was determined to bring order to the hospital wards on her appointment as superintendent of nurses in 1911. She did—and unleashed a torrent of complaints and criticisms from the medical interns, the visiting physicians, the nursing staff, and the nursing students. She was, it seemed, treating house staff with little or no respect. She displayed an "absence of decorum and attention" to other physicians. Her supervisory staff of trained nurses complained about her "autocratic manner" and her practice of rebuking them in front of students and orderlies. Her students were "nervous and unhappy" about her orders to perform "indelicate procedures" on male patients. Indeed, never, in the eyes of visiting physicians, had the quality of nursing care sunk so low.[20]

If discipline was the cornerstone of the day-to-day formative experiences that transformed women into trained nurses, the day-to-day encounters among nursing supervisors, attending physicians, nursing students, and medical interns at Grady provide a rare glimpse of the complex realities surrounding the creation of such experiences. Certainly, hierarchical lines of authority remained important. But they were not sacrosanct. They existed within a political world in which open criticisms and alliances of the relatively powerless—in particular, those between nursing students and medical interns—proved to be effective ways to circumvent the prerogatives of department heads and to place some checks on abuses of power. They were situated within a racialized world where white concerns about propriety had to be seriously addressed.

These lines of authority also played out within a social world that needed order rather than turmoil, contentment rather than demoralization, and good publicity rather than scandalous press. Reports of drunken house staff and unhappy nurses undercut the message of hope and progress that the hospital hoped to deliver to a city still suspicious about the need for municipal support for the sick poor.[21] And inside the institution, such reports spread disillusionment, disappointment, and the defection of skilled nurses in an already short-staffed, resource-starved, and somewhat suspect environment.[22]

Feebeck, in fact, struggled to learn the cardinal commandment of running a nurses training program: Thou shall keep thy nurses reasonably happy. Her white students were not happy—and they were not powerless. Some simply left training.[23] Others joined with the hospital's medical interns and went straight to the governing medical board of the institution with their concerns. By 1913 the board, feeling "harassed" by the constant complaints of poor treatment from student nurses and interns, launched a formal investigation. It uncovered a training school experience that exemplified all the worst aspects of an emphasis on disciplined performance. It found instances where a student was forced to work for twenty-seven hours straight as a punishment for carelessness. It documented another of a student kept continuously on an isolation case until she fainted from exhaustion. Only four of the thirty students in the school felt they could approach their superintendent with any question or concern. And none of the house staff felt they were treated with any semblance of common courtesy.[24]

The board debated what to do. Some members called for Feebeck's immediate dismissal. Her behavior bordered on criminal, and it seemed to explain the lack of applicants to the training school. Others felt that Feebeck had done good work reorganizing the training school. She had introduced the first three-year nurses training program in Georgia, allowing Grady to boast, in theory if not in fact, of providing an educational experience similar to that in northern training schools. They also believed it would be problematic if staff thought they could go over the head of their respective departments and straight to governing boards with their complaints. Still, they acknowledged, the fact that so few of Feebeck's nurses felt they could approach her indicated serious problems. They reached a compromise. Feebeck could remain as superintendent if she agreed to a public humiliation by writing a letter of apology to her staff.

She did. It is true, she admitted, that some students were denied time off or refused permission to leave the hospital without any explanations as to why. In the future, she promised, students would receive that information. In retrospect, she acknowledged, she had meted out excessive and extreme punishment, and she would change this error. She felt it "unfortunate" that some saw her as unapproachable and unwilling to listen to explanations about particular acts or behavior. She would, she assured them, work to "banish" that impression, listen to her students, and give all reprimands in private. But she also wanted her staff to know why she did what she did.

Feebeck knew she had the privilege of race within the Grady. But she was also well aware that its prerogatives stopped at the hospital's doors. She recognized that the idea of white trained nursing in the South remained problematic when images of nurses were framed by the traditions of care by African American slaves. To her chagrin, her own white students were still denied the seemingly self-evident and chivalrous protection of a separate residence, not only because of a decision to spend resources elsewhere but also because such decisions reflected the lingering conflation of their work with that as easily done by African American men and women. Manners and morals would be these women's strongest defense. Your reputation, Feebeck reminded her staff and students, is your "stock in trade." And the result of her emphasis on discipline "is a reputation of those who graduate here that is not equaled by those of any other institution in this part of the country."[25] Feebeck promised "civility" and, by all accounts, delivered it as well.[26]

African American Nurses at Grady

Feebeck's promise of civility, however, did not extend to the African American wards at Grady. By 1914 an earlier experiment employing trained African American nurses had evolved into a plan to provide formal training to them.[27] Ludie Andrews, a 1906 graduate of the Spelman Nurses Training School, assumed responsibility for the education, the supervision, and the care delivered by these women. Andrews came with strong credentials: she had experience in private duty, caring for white patients in the same typhoid epidemic that had drawn Van de Vrede to the city from her home in Wisconsin. She had served as the superintendent of the Lula Grove Hospital and Training School, a small Atlanta hospital established by white physicians for African American patients. And she was determined to make her African American training school one of the most prestigious in the state.

As in the North, racialized lines of authority remained important in a context where markers of social stratification needed to be as clear as those of physical segregation. Andrews' position could not be conflated with Feebeck's. Although Andrews considered herself as the "superintendent" of the African American training school, she knew that the white medical committee to which she reported consistently referred to her as its "head nurse." Andrews' ambition was to have her school recognized as an accredited training school by Georgia's Board of Examiners, the newly formed state agency charged with establishing educational standards for the state's training schools. Andrews achieved this goal in 1920. But it came only after careful negotiations ensured that Grady's African American graduates would never be confused with its white ones. African American trained students and graduate nurses would wear different uniforms, caps, and pins signifying their association, not with Grady Hospital per se, but with the newly chartered and separately titled "Municipal Training School for Colored Nurses."[28]

But such racialized lines were also not sacrosanct. To underscore the seriousness of her plans for the African American training school on her arrival at Grady in 1914, Andrews and her students refused to assume responsibility for the care of African American patients until they received assurances from the white medical board "that they would not be wasting their time" and working, as they had in the past, for a certificate rather than the more prestigious diploma that Grady's white graduates received. But Andrews found that the disciplined and hierarchical lines of authority she hoped to establish within her world existed within realities every bit as complex as those that had been experienced by Feebeck. Her students, displeased with the disciplinary outcome of an altercation between an orderly and a particular student, staged a fifteen-minute work stoppage when, unlike their white counterparts, they could not get an immediate hearing with the white medical board. The board quickly arranged a meeting. And Andrews immediately added an additional week to their service before graduation to reassert her authority.[29]

Neither Andrews nor Feebeck ever lost sight of the fact that their ambitions for themselves, their students, and their training schools lay within a broader racialized context. Andrews remained grateful to white physicians who provided her with opportunities to prove her ability. She also realized that their help was part of a deeply engrained process that normalized segregation by demonstrating instances of fair and equal, albeit separate, experiences to those on the other side of the color line. But she recognized the possibilities of holding such white colleagues to their vision of their society as fair, separate, and equal. Much to the chagrin of white nurses like Feebeck, who were determined that the title "registered nurse" would only refer to the best-educated among themselves, Andrews mobilized her white male supporters in a battle for the right to take the licensure exam necessary to become a registered nurse.

The Battle over Registration

Registration battles flared across the country in the early twentieth century as small groups of trained nurses in every state sought the same legal protections for their practice of nursing that physicians had for their practice of medicine. Since they had no control over the training school experiences offered by individual hospitals, these women hoped that creating mandatory state licensure standards for postgraduate practice would add the force of law to their tireless promotion of their voluntary standards. If, they reasoned, only graduates of training programs who met certain criteria could take licensing exams, and if, as they hoped, patients, hospitals, and other health care agencies recognized only licensed or "registered" nurses as fully trained ones, then nurses could force the closure of small and specialized hospitals and require substantive improvements in the curricular offerings and clinical experiences in most others. But administrators of these small and specialized hospitals, who valued the care students in their training schools brought to their patients, and the graduates of such programs, who strongly believed in their work and the worth of their nursing diploma, fought back. In state after state, well into the 1930s, licensure require-ments remained voluntary, and only some hospitals, the military, and public health agencies required such credentials for employment.

If not necessary, licensure and the accompanying right to the title registered nurse were self-consciously constructed as prestigious. The exact standards for such credentialing varied from state to state, reflect-ing the inevitable political compromises among nurses, hospital admin-istrators, and physicians from different backgrounds and with different interests. But they remained deliberately exclusionary, since only some nurses in any given state could attest to meeting licensing standards.[30] Some African American nurses in the other northern, midwestern, and southern states had met these standards and had received the appropri-ate credentials. Ludie Andrews sought to make it possible for African American nurses in Georgia to do the same.

The white leaders of the Georgia State Nurses Association (GSNA), formed in 1907 to organize the push for state registration, were deter-mined that Andrews would not win this right. In their minds, nursing licensure would finally disentangle their state's particularly compli-cated associations among class and race. Like all other southern as-sociations, the GSNA refused membership to African American nurses. But it was much more adamant than most southern state nurses asso-ciations in its position that such nurses could not become licensed—that there would be no means that might create any semblance of repre-sentations of equality between white and African American nurses. It established its own two-class system in which properly credentialed white graduates would receive a license to practice as registered nurses, and similarly credentialed African American graduates would receive certificates only attesting to their training.[31] Historian Carla Schissel has painted a vivid picture of the multiple meanings of the threat that Ludie Andrews' application presented to the GSNA. It would strengthen associations between nursing and African American and white do-mestic service. It would create nightmares about racial mixing as African American nurses competed with white ones. And it would so-lidify the use of race as an effective tool that outsiders would use to challenge the ambitions of those who believed in the possibilities of trained nursing.[32] It would be, in the end, a wedge that would destroy a carefully laid but still fragile plan to appropriate the identity of a trained nurse as the prerogative of white, middle-class women in Georgia.

The GSNA's public comments framed the issues surrounding its persistent refusal of Andrews' application as a commitment to high educational standards that had nothing to do with race. When necessary, it pointed to its 1912 registration of Mattie Madora White, a graduate of New York City's Lincoln Hospital Training School.[33] But Andrews, with influential support from some in the white and African American medical communities, reframed the issue as "racial prejudice" that now involved not only her but all African American nurses in Georgia who graduated from schools that met the state's own standards. There is some evidence that the GSNA may have been willing to grant Andrews' request as an exceptional request by an exceptional individual.[34] But the GSNA felt it had to harden its position when it became clear that Andrews' quest was to broaden her application to represent the legitimate aspirations of all qualified African American nurses.

The GSNA took an untenable position and held firmly to it until 1919.[35] It had the public support to do so. Georgia, the most populous southern state, was also the state with the highest number of African American residents who seemed to threaten white supremacy. Its politicians blatantly manipulated white fear of African American achievement. It remained one of the most racially violent of all the southern states with the highest lynching rates of any state until well after World War I. It struggled with ways to make sense of the growing numbers of working-class white women migrating to its urban mills, factories, and offices seeking gainful employment. Furthermore, Georgia's white nurses knew of and resented their somewhat suspect place in wider world of northern nursing. Georgia-born Dorothy Barfield, in New York City for postgraduate education, remembered feeling horrified as one instructor criticized southern nurses as "lazy and stupid" and as another announced her determination to break her of her southern accent. But Georgia's nurses also had no use for northerners who presumed to tell them what to do. "All right, you damn Yankee," one such nurse told Helen Smith when she tried to hold an integrated class with white and African American students, "have you got your ticket back north?"[36]

The Work of Georgia's Nurses

This animosity took place against a backdrop of limited employment prospects for white and African American training school graduates in the South. Theoretically, most opportunities for work would be in the private duty labor market, where one nurse would care for one sick patient at home or, increasingly, through the 1920s, in a hospital. Some such prospects existed, particularly in urban areas like Atlanta, with a growing number of middle-class families who could afford such admittedly expensive care. But given southern traditions of care by slave women, both white and African American nurses competed for these opportunities with invariably white families. By the 1920s the urban southern private duty labor market, like its northern counterparts, had become hopelessly overcrowded as steady streams of young training school graduates competed for limited employment opportunities with their older nursing colleagues. "I hate to seem inhospitable in not wanting more nurses," one Georgia nurse wrote in response to a national survey of postgraduate employment options, "but we are already overcrowded, and it makes me miserable as we cannot all keep busy here."[37]

Some other opportunities existed in Georgia's slowly developing public health system. The state's fiercely independent counties had long traditions of resistance to what they saw as outside interference in their right to take care of their own needs and to the increases in taxes that might support state interventions. It had as long a tradition of refusing to acknowledge the seriousness of illness and disability related to malaria, hookworm, pellagra, tuberculosis, and maternal morbidity. It also had a sharp resentment of outsiders—of both northern philanthropists and the federal government who tried to address its health problems.[38] But the persistent and successful crusades by private foundations and public agencies had some successes. The Rosenwald Foundation encouraged education. Moreover, the Rockefeller Foundation's campaign to conquer hookworm and malaria and the federal Public Health Service's interest in eradicating pellagra nourished a nascent, albeit rudimentary, public health movement in Georgia.[39] However, the state remained overwhelmingly poor and rural. In 1930, for example, approximately 130 counties still had no money to support any kind of public health initiative.[40]

In Georgia, the role of the public health nurse mirrored that of the public health system: small, underdeveloped, and underfunded. Atlanta had the state's first public health nurses. In 1911, the city hired such women to look after the health of its children in schools. All white schools had their own individual nurses. One African American nurse, Charity Collins, took care of all the students in all the city's segregated African American schools.[41] The role came slowly to other parts of the state with the federal monies that accompanied the 1921 Sheppard-Towner Act, a federal program designed to provide health care and education to women and children. The monies allowed the hiring of one white public health nurse, and in 1923 a donation from the Methodist Woman's Missionary Society provided for the employment of an African American one. But this program proved unsustainable. The Sheppard-Towner Act required state matching funds, and Georgia only matched $5,000 of the $19,000 in matching funds available.[42] State, county, and municipal agencies provided other sources of employment, but these were scarce. In 1931, Georgia ranked 38th out of 46 states in terms of the numbers of public health nurses per capita. Thirty-two agencies provided employment for only 151 nurses, primarily within boards of health, tuberculosis control associations, and insurance company nursing organizations. Of these nurses, 30 percent worked in Atlanta, and fully 80 percent worked in the state's largest cities.[43]

But if opportunities for employment as public health nurses remained limited at the start of the state's initiatives, they deteriorated in the economic ravages of the 1930s. By 1933, only four public health nurses remained employed by state agencies. By 1935, the few opportunities for paid public health nursing work came through the federal Works Projects Administration and, after 1936, through Federal Social Security Health Funds, which provided care to the aged, the unemployed, and dependent children through a state director, assistant director, and eighteen field nurses.[44]

African American public health nurses represented almost 30 percent of Georgia's public health nurses.[45] These positions were extraordinarily competitive. In 1937, for example, there were fifty applicants for two public health nursing positions that had become available in Atlanta.[46] These were almost exclusively centered in urban areas where population numbers could support the employment of a nurse for each race. If there were to be any public health nurse in any of the poorer and more rural counties, it would be a white nurse. White southerners had grown up with traditions that allowed them to accept the physical care of African American nurses. But these same traditions of mastery, dominance, and white supremacy meant they would not countenance the idea that these African American women might know more than they did and that they might be able to actually teach them about health and hygiene.

Furthermore, unlike in the North, where salary differentials were more moderate, African American salaries were substantially less than their white counterparts. In 1925, for example, the Georgia State Board of Health paid white nurses $200 per month and African American nurses only $150. And African American nurses had no opportunities for advancement. When the nursing director of Atlanta's Anti-Tuberculosis Association (which paid white and African American nurses $125 and $80 respectively) was asked about the possibility of promotion for African American nurses, she tersely replied: "None whatsoever."[47]

The Lives of Georgia's Nurses

Georgia's more rural counties held some other opportunities. But many white and African American nurses had grown up in such places, and to them, nurses training was a way to create a different kind of life.[48] Beatrice Parramore, a white nurse, grew up on a farm in Worth County and, after high school, had worked in a dime store in the nearby town of Sylvester. But, she remembered, she worked there only long enough to realize that was not what she wanted to do for the rest of her life. Her cousin was a nurse and seemed to have constructed a good life. So even though Parramore had never been in a hospital and had no idea what went on in one, she enrolled in the Macon Hospital Training School for Nurses in Macon, Georgia, in 1930. Similarly, Magnolia Brown, an African American nurse from rural Stevens County, had spent her childhood summers living with an aunt in Atlanta. "When you see all the advantages there," she remembered, "you just don't want to go back." She lived with her aunt through high school before enrolling in the Lamar School of Nursing in Augusta, the African American counterpart to the Augusta Hospital's School of Nursing for white women.[49]

Some nurses remembered encouragement from their families for their ambitions to train as nurses. Pauline English, a white nurse born in the small town of Covington in Newton County, remembered her mother investigating the possibility of nurses training schools for her daughters because there were "no opportunities" for women in their region of the state. Mamie Lee Miller Wilson's grandmother fought to get her admitted to the African American training school at Grady in 1938. Grady at that time required all applicants to have a degree from one of the state's accredited high schools. It had refused Wilson's admission because her segregated Savannah high school could not meet accreditation standards. Her grandmother was furious. She took Wilson's application straight to the state's Board of Education. Her granddaughter, she argued, took full advantage of the only schools the state had seen fit to make available to African American women in that city, and it was unfair that she would then be denied admission to a nurses training school. She asked the board to find a solution to this dilemma—and it did. Wilson attended Grady.[50]

Laverne Johnson always wanted to be a nurse: as a young white child, she had been impressed with the fact that a nurse she knew drove a model A automobile. That, she remembered, "was the height of my ambition." But many others, like their counterparts throughout the country, saw nursing as an alternative to dreams of college and careers that they could not afford. Elizabeth Horne, an African American nurse from rural Hawkinsville in Pulaski county, Georgia, had wanted to teach. But after a boll weevil infestation destroyed her family's cotton crop, she could no longer depend on their financial support while she earned her certificate. Nursing was a more reasonable alternative, and she saw nothing but a future of marriage and farming if she remained home. The fact that nurses training schools in Georgia charged no tuition and, in fact, offered a stipend attracted women who wanted to create a life different from the one they had known. Still, it sometimes required a leap of faith. Alice Latham Herndon, for example, wanted to attend college like her white parents had, but in 1934 her family had few resources. At the young age of sixteen, she entered training even though she did not know a thing about the field and struggled with the fact that it seemed more like domestic service. It was, she remembered, "considered a more menial type of work than a profession."[51]

Given the conflation of nursing and working-class domestic service, many more white than African American women remembered their families' dismay about their wish to train as nurses. Theodora Floyd remembered the "bombshell" she dropped on her parents when she announced her wish to train as a nurse. She wanted to serve as a missionary in China, and she decided that her chances of selection would be greater with a background as a nurse rather than as a teacher. Bessie May Dickey wanted to train as a nurse, but her father insisted on college. Her mother, who had died when she was five, was a college graduate and a teacher, and he wanted his daughter to be one as well. Dickey tried college, was miserable, and eventually entered the Annie Mills Archibold Training School for Nurses in Thomasville even though, she reported, "my family thought that nursing was just one of the lowest grade professions you could do."[52]

Certainly, northern-trained nurses also struggled with the public's often problematic perception of their practice. Nurses' engagement with medical knowledge and their formation of an identity in the crucible of the training experience looked inward toward their own sense of themselves as practitioners. They remained largely invisible to those whose experience of nurses and nursing remained centered only around the intimate body work necessary in the care of the sick and to those who never witnessed their independent and skillful responses to medical emergencies. In Georgia, those white and African American women who felt most supported in their decisions about training as nurses came from families with aunts, sisters, or cousins who had also entered nursing and who had a more direct experience with the range of the work and its worth. Ruth Melber, for example, came from what she described as an African American "family of nurses." And Lemma Athena Mosley Williamson's grandmother, mother, aunt, and two cousins all trained as nurses at the Hall Chaudron Training School in a small, private white hospital near their home in Cedarton, Georgia.[53]

The invisibility of the real work and worth of nursing was also complicated by the fact that nursing and domestic service were the few kinds of work in the South that easily crossed carefully constructed color lines. There existed traditions in which it was acceptable for African American women to care for white patients and for white women to care for African American patients. Nillar Orander Almond remembered a "colored nurse" from Columbia who took care of her white nephew when she was a child. And Birdie Torrance McFarlin had similar memories of a white nurse who took care of her after her broken leg. Such care had always carried different meanings and existed within different rituals of deference and obligation. But, increasingly, African American women appropriated parts of the work of nursing to enhance their own place within service traditions. Often it was as formally trained nurses that they served in ways that reworked the traditions of slavery. In fact, one such Atlanta nurse explained, white families were finding it increasingly "fashionable" to turn to African American trained nurses rather than servants as their young children's maids.[54]

Unlike in the North, Georgia's white trained nurses had few visible and public examples of respected and respectable white women choosing to do the work of nursing. They did have some. Rosalie Howell, whose father bought a controlling interest in the *Atlanta Constitution* in 1901 and edited it through 1936, served as a nurse during World War I. Her letters to her family from the battlefields of France, reprinted in the *Constitution,* were full of the commitment and the war-time drama that only female nurses could experience.[55] Howell did not remain connected to nursing's cause, but Nell Kendall Hodgson did. Hodgson, the daughter of a prominent Georgia family, had started nurses' training at St. Mary's Hospital in Athens in 1910, but she left before graduation to marry Robert Woodruff, an Atlanta businessman who would soon make Coca-Cola a national and later an international symbol. As Mrs. Robert Woodruff, she played an important and visible role in recruiting and training Georgia women to serve as nurses aides for the American Red Cross during World War I. Woodruff respected the education and the work of formally trained nurses and remained involved with nursing after the war. But other social commitments limited the scope of her involvement to Atlanta's Emory University, the site of significant Woodruff philanthropy, and its Hospital Training School for Nurses.[56]

Northern nurses, with good cause, complained about the lack of broad social support for their agenda of reforming the care of the sick in homes and in hospitals. But they did find some sympathetic ears. Influential white women often championed the cause of public health nursing. The Carnegie and the Rockefeller Foundations invested some money in nursing education, and by 1923 there were four freestanding baccalaureate programs in nursing. More and more larger urban hospitals, seeking to maintain prestigious positions, had added two additional years at associated colleges and universities for those nurses wishing to complete the requirements for a bachelor's degree after they finished a traditional three-year hospital-based program.

There were few such advanced educational programs in the South. "Someone," one southern nurse hoped in 1933, "is going to talk loud enough for the public to hear that the education of the Nurse is the responsibility of the community and not the burden of the sick public."[57] There also seemed few voices in support of southern nurses even within the national nursing community. The internal national nursing critique of the late 1920s was that there were both too many nurses with inadequate pre-training backgrounds and training school experiences and too few who could meet the demands of the modern health care environment. Southern nurses knew that this was directed at many of their own experiences in states with a poorly developed public school systems and with a preponderance of small hospital training schools offering valuable but limited clinical experiences.[58] White southern nurses also confronted the problematic issue of being from a region that boasted the dubious distinction of having the highest number of married white women in the nursing workforce. Thirty-three percent of southern married women remained in the workforce in the late 1920s, well above both the national average of 20 percent and the 18 percent benchmark set by white northeastern nurses.[59] African American women were expected to work after marriage. White women were not.

Race and Place

Georgia's white nurses, without substantive backing from middle-class supporters and with a sense of their own uneasy place in Georgia's social order, chose instead to reinforce associations based on the privileges of race. They ensured that both had separate work spaces in public health agencies that employed white and African American nurses. These spaces often located African American nurses' offices in basements. In situations of unavoidable contact, such as meetings held within these agencies, African American nurses sat in the back of the room and took part in discussions only if explicitly called upon to do so.[60] More pointedly, white nurses in Georgia ensured they would be addressed with the honorific of "Miss" or "Mrs.," while their African American counterparts would be addressed by their first name only. They denied African American nurses the title of "nurse," although the racial distinction between "Miss" or "Mrs." for white nurses and "nurse" for African American ones was accepted practice in other parts of the country. African American nurses resented the vehemence with which white nurses worked to make sure there would be no social or professional equality between the races. But, as Lena LaVette pointed out, protests would have lead to dismissal from much-needed jobs. She had her own way of handling this issue. She tried to make sure all her conversations with white colleagues were structured in such a way that she never had to use any titles.[61]

White nurses in Georgia continued to complain about their inability to secure legislation that would mandate strict educational entrance standards to their training schools and a comprehensive program of content and clinical experiences before graduation. But by 1935, they had secured mandatory licensing laws with criteria that sharply curtailed the number of small nurses training schools in the state. The numbers of training schools in Georgia decreased from 35 in 1920 to 32 in 1930, and then plummeted to 16 by 1936. White nursing leaders succeeded by creating strategic alliances with surgeons and representative medical associations looking toward the prestigious accreditation of their particular hospitals by the American College of Surgeons. They publicly framed their achievements as that of forcing hospitals to recognize their inability to offer sound educational programs for would-be nurses. But amidst the hard economic realities of the 1930s, they privately emphasized that unless educational standards reflected national norms, Georgia-trained nurses would not be allowed to practice in other states. And without the possibility of geographic mobility, potential nursing students—still the lifeblood of hospital nursing care—would look for other kinds of opportunities elsewhere.[62]

These new licensing laws affected the choices available to many of Georgia's rural women. But these laws had an even more devastating impact on the viability of the training schools run in small African American–controlled hospitals. The economic catastrophe of the 1930s hit these training programs and hospitals hard as many found themselves without the financial resources to continue. By the mid-1930s there were no longer any African American–controlled training schools for nurses in the state. The four of the five training schools that continued to offer opportunities to African American women in Georgia were in large urban hospitals that ran separate white and African American training programs, controlled by white nursing superintendents.[63] Spelman's McVicar Hospital Training School for Nurses, the first training school for nurses in the state, achieved accreditation by the Georgia State Board of Nursing, but its student nurses, like its medical students and staff, remained under the supervision of white clinicians.

As Darlene Clark Hine has shown, many northern African American hospitals and training schools survived the economic ravages of the 1930s because of the social and material support that middle-class African American club and church women provided.[64] Georgia had such active and influential African American women.[65] In Atlanta, Lugenia Burns Hope's Atlanta Neighborhood Union was the most visible and effective of private African American women's organizations dedicated to strengthening its community. It had begun as a collective gathering of Hope's neighbors and fellow faculty wives at Spelman and Atlanta Baptist Colleges. Their initial goal was to address the appalling lack of recreational facilities for their children. By the 1930s, the gathering had become a powerful and organized settlement house reaching all of Atlanta's black neighborhoods and acclaimed as a national and international role model for community organization. It took the health of Atlanta's African American community as one of its primary concerns. It established an outpatient clinic that provided medical and nursing care. It led city-wide vaccination campaigns. It brought classes on health, hygiene, and proper mothering into the city's African American churches.[66] It also sponsored Atlanta's participation in the annual National Negro Health Week, a powerful vehicle for personal and political persuasion in a place where African Americans lacked legal rights.[67]

Ludie Andrews worked for the Neighborhood Union after leaving Grady, giving health and hygiene lectures in Atlanta's African American public schools, churches, and private homes and participating in the formal educational activities of its National Negro Health Week.[68] The Neighborhood Union employed and valued the work of trained nurses, but it, as well as other African American women's organizations, provided little support to those who wanted to be nurses. Some African

American church women did take an interest in the welfare of black children at Grady, making plans each Christmas to make sure that they had toys, but African American women reformers, like their white counterparts, seemed to concentrate their resources on other causes and left the hospital-based training system in the hands of white administrators, physicians, and nurses. It is not at all clear that their support, even if offered, would have been accepted. Annie Bess Feebeck remained as superintendent of both the white and African American training schools through the 1930s, and even the white women in the Hospital's Aid Association feared her wrath. The Grady Aid Association had changed its name to the "Auxiliary," in 1931, and it reiterated that its purpose was "charity." That charity, the by-laws continued, was to be delivered "in friendly and helpful relations with nurses . . . and without interference in hospital routine and with no unnecessary visiting in the wards."[69] But the end result of decisions by African American club and church women to focus on other reform possibilities was the abandonment of Georgia's African American nursing students to separate and unequal resources and to the racism of their white supervisors.

White Supervisors and African American Students

Ethel Johns painted a vivid picture of what Grady's African American students faced under Feebeck's tenure. Johns had been commissioned by the Rockefeller Foundation in 1925 to survey the educational opportunities available to women in African American nursing schools throughout the United States. The report would serve as a basis for any future decisions about how the foundation might best concentrate its considerable education and public health philanthropy. Edwin Embree, the director of the Rockefeller Foundation's studies, suggested that Johns concentrate on a number of leading African American training schools. He wanted her to visit Atlanta, but he also warned her against thinking that the foundation might see any hope in investing there. The city, he noted was a "bad center" of race relations and a site where there had always been only "bitterness and bad blood."[70]

Even with this warning, Johns was shocked when she entered what was then known as the "Colored Division of the Grady Hospital." The hospital itself, converted from an old and dilapidated medical school, was "forbidding," "forlorn," and "evil smelling." Segregation was such that even African American interns were not allowed on African American wards. The inability to gain any systematic clinical experience put such medical students at a distinct disadvantage not only in relation to their white medical peers but, just as importantly, to African American nursing students who could claim what they could not: real clinical knowledge and skills honed through months and years of practice. "We envy the nurses," a medical student told Johns. "They at least get a chance—we get none"[71]

The chance came at a high cost. African American student nurses lived in the hospital. Four slept in one room so small that the beds were almost touching each other; <u>sixteen</u> night nurses, Johns underscored, slept in two rooms in the basement in a "fetid" atmosphere. The work of these women on the hospital's wards seemed to lack "finish," Johns wrote, and there seemed a distinct absence of "niceties" such as privacy for women in labor. But she admired the care they gave their patients. "There was an energetic air about the whole place," she reported, "which gave one the idea that in the main the work was somehow done and reasonably good care given."[72]

Feebeck, described by Johns as a "woman of considerable force," admitted frank contempt for all "niggers." Johns suspected she did have a "sneaking regard for the colored students," but her opinions of them so virulently reflected the racist discourse of the period that Johns departed from her usual custom of recording only summary statements after school visits. She felt she had to list these opinions verbatim in Feebeck's "own terse English." The African American students were, Feebeck had told Johns, "such liars"; "they shift responsibility whenever they can"; "they quarrel constantly among themselves and will cut up each others clothes for spite"; "unless they are constantly watched they will steal anything in sight"; "most of them haven't any morals." Still, Johns concluded, even Feebeck had to eventually acknowledge that "there are some fine girls among them, good nurses, splendid with the patients."[73]

Unlike peers at African American–owned hospitals and training schools who worked with and for African American physicians, nurses, and patients, those at Grady had little protection from the day-to-day assaults on their competence and character from white supervisors and instructors. In addition, they tended to be young. Lena LaVette lied about her age to gain admission at seventeen.[74] But LaVette may not have needed to lie. In most cases, and as long as they met the requisite educational requirements (albeit lower than those of their white student counterparts), white superintendents of nursing preferred younger African American students to older ones. Younger students, Johns heard over and over again from white superintendents, were less likely than older ones to challenge the terms of their treatment.[75] But if reluctant to directly confront their treatment and risk expulsion from an education that would increase their social and financial opportunities, African American students seemed constantly aware of it. Many, Birdie Torrance McFarlin recalled, were simply waiting for graduation, when they would take the first train north, often to Harlem Hospital in New York City. There were few illusions about racial equality in the northern United States. Roberta Roberts Spencer's sister worked in New York City. Restaurants there, she reported, would serve an African American customer. But as soon as that customer left, staff would return to the kitchen and break the plate upon which the meal had been served.[76] In the North, there only seemed more opportunity for employment and better wages.

In many respects, those white and African American nurses who remained in Georgia had much in common in this particular world. They both struggled to find support for the legitimacy of their practice in a place reluctant to assume any substantive public responsibility for the care of the sick poor. They occupied a tenuous place in a political and social system that remained deeply suspicious of the publicly supported hospitals and public health care systems in which they worked. Georgia's African American student nurses suffered from the same absence of lay supporters that white nursing students also experienced. They both struggled to gain support for genteel nurses' homes rather than sterile dormitories or unused patient rooms. In the South, and in a world where the care of the sick for pay remained within the realm of private domestic service, separate nurses' homes were only grudgingly granted white women who would train as nurses, and only rarely granted African American ones.

In Georgia, both white and African American women lived and worked in a place where they had to constantly negotiate and reappropriate ideas about properly racialized social spaces in their wish for an authoritative voice in the care of the sick. They struggled to gain support from their respective communities as they tried to appropriate new identities that challenged assumptions about their work. Without such support, neither group could call upon the privileges of class to support their ideas and the work and worth of trained nurses.

White nurses were advantaged in that they held the privilege of race. They constructed meanings around racialized nursing identities by looking inward to the norms of their own local communities. African American nurses, by contrast, had to look outward to the experiences of other professional friends in Georgia and more national networks outside the state in their quest to achieve some semblance of equal, albeit separate, recognition. Their struggle against the privileges of white supremacy lasted longer than those in any other state. The Georgia State Nurses Association was the last state association to officially desegregate. It did so in 1961 only after the American Nurses Association threatened to expel Georgia from the national organization if it failed to do so.

CHAPTER 6

A Tale of Two Associations

White and African American Nurses in North Carolina

I N 1946, THE SEGREGATED BOARDS of both the American Nurses Association (ANA) and the National Association of Colored Graduate Nurses (NACGN) endorsed the principle of one integrated professional association fighting for the rights, the respect, the prerogatives, and the privileges of all registered nurses in the United States. Both boards linked this principle to that of the war that had engulfed them, their constituents, their country, and the world. In the midst of the raging struggle for the survival of democratic principles, they asserted, American nurses had to pledge commitment to the equality that was at the core of such principles. They also had to assume leadership in race relations among all professional medical organizations and eliminate all remaining barriers to the complete integration of nurses into all levels of professional organizations, training schools and universities, and hospitals and health care agencies. Dr. Montague Cobb, the editor of the *Journal of the National Medical Association,* also applauded this position, noting that it served as a not-so-subtle rebuke of the "do-nothing" policy of the American Medical Association.[1]

These high ideals had a history. For decades, coalitions of progressive and largely northern-based African American and white nurses had worked together with prominent lay advocates and philanthropists to slowly but steadily broaden educational and practice opportunities for African American nurses. The National Organization for Public Health Nursing (NOPHN) had provided the administrative linchpin. Founded in 1912 to represent the interests of public health and public health nursing, NOPHN had always encouraged African American membership. By the 1930s, organizational grants from the Rosenwald and the Rockefeller Foundations and individual contributions from philanthropists such as Frances Payne Bolton had allowed it to move the idea of integrating all American nursing organizations to the forefront of its political agenda. Simultaneously, educational fellowships from the foundations provided the opportunity for a small number of African American nurses to gain postgraduate collegiate education and to re-emerge with white colleagues as a new generation of American nursing leaders. These leaders were politically connected, savvy, single-minded, and ambitious. As the United States prepared for entry into World War II, they set their sights on destroying the Jim Crow policies that had historically excluded African American nurses from military service. Their moment came in early 1945, when then-President Franklin Roosevelt announced his support for legislation that would draft white nurses to meet the army's overwhelming needs. The ensuing public outrage at the deliberate exclusion of qualified African American nurses from voluntary military service was at once entirely spontaneous and carefully orchestrated. It quickly led to the landmark 1945 presidential order that officially desegregated nursing in the U.S. Armed Services.[2]

But by the late 1940s these ideals were matched with concrete actions by the largest American nursing organization, the ANA, which had long purported to represent more than just a specialized and progressive few. By 1949, African American nurses occupied positions on key ANA committees. An interracial study group had worked out the details about how the ANA would absorb the professional, economic, and social functions that the National Association of Colored Graduate Nurses had long provided to its members. On January 26, 1951—with great fanfare—the NACGN formally dissolved. This was a nationally recognized event. Eleanor Roosevelt, an outspoken advocate of civil rights and a critical voice in the campaign to desegregate her late husband's military and medical services, sent her "warm congratulations" from her new position as head of the United Nations Human Rights Commission. Ralph Bunche, the noted African American diplomat and UN ambassador who had just received the Noble Peace Prize for his work negotiating an armistice between the Israelis and the Palestinians, noted the "signal contribution" that nursing in general, and the NACGN in particular, had made toward realizing the dream of a day "when all minority peoples in this great nation will be fully integrated and fully treated as equals."[3]

Above all, wrote Mabel Staupers, the former NACGN's executive secretary and future member of the ANA's Board of Directors, the idea of one association representing all American nurses irrespective of race, religion, or ethnicity represented a leap "of great faith." Staupers, a tiny bundle of energy, intelligence, fearlessness, and political savvy, was one of the most important architects of nursing's desegregation strategy. In 1951, the NAACP awarded her its prestigious Spingarn Medal in recognition of her role "in realizing the full integration of Negro nursing into the organized ranks of the nursing profession in this country."[4] But Staupers and her African American and white colleagues clearly understood that the desegregation of the ANA marked only the beginning, not the end, of the battle for the professional integration of nursing. State associations—not individual nurses—were the ANA's constituent members, and the national policy was immediately contested by state associations in the American south. Battle lines had already been drawn in many southern states even as the national celebrations began.

This chapter explores the dimensions of this struggle for desegregation among nurses in North Carolina, one of the few southern states with extant records of active, albeit segregated, white and African American state nurses associations. North Carolina was, in fact, one of the more progressive states in the ANA's Southern Division. Unlike in Georgia, for example, white and African American nurses in North Carolina had always taken the same registration exam. Certainly, many North Carolinians shared with Georgians similar assumptions about the work and worth of those who cared for the sick for money. But the impact of these assumptions were moderated by the state's stronger sense of its public responsibility to the poor and its greater willingness to invest in an educational and public health infrastructure. North Carolina also had a reasonably strong commitment to a fair allocation of state, federal, and philanthropic educational and public health dollars to its African American as well as its white citizens. It had a history of being among the first southern states to employ at least some African American dentists and public health nurses as an integral part of its state and county maternal, infant, and school health work.[5]

Not surprisingly, the stories told by white and African American North Carolina nurses placed the nurses themselves within their state's southern progressive traditions. White nurses in the North Carolina State Nurses Association (NCSNA) still basked in their state's reputation as a place of harmonious race relations respectful of law, tradition, and "social custom," while African American nurses in the State Association of Negro Registered Nurses (SANRN) clung to ideas of equality and to the political strategies and compromises necessary to make these ideas a reality. But as this chapter argues, more private stories told in oral histories and organizational records help up us move beyond public rhetoric. These stories give voice to particular assumptions, expectations, and experiences. They show how nursing—as an identity, a professionalized idea, and a practice discipline—existed within more complicated relationships than just those of their own particular communities of class, race, place. It also existed within highly gendered and equally racialized and classed relationships with other social groups, with medicine, with academia, and with their national associations. And this ability to look out—to look to the politics, the practices, the animating ideas, and the social realities of groups other than their own—helped nurses, albeit sometimes reluctantly, to incorporate changing ideas and ideals into their social as well as professional identities. In North Carolina, it allowed white and African American nurses to come together around powerful ideas about class and professionalism, if not around the realities of race and desegregated practice.

The Idea of Professionalism

Both white and African American nursing leaders were committed to using the idea of professionalism to challenge the social and racialized stereotypes that often compromised their claims to power and authority in the care of the sick. Such an idea emphasized gendered dynamics, highlighting women's role in the care of the sick. But it simultaneously surrounded this role with carefully constructed forms of disciplined, dispassionate practice long claimed by the powerful world of white male privilege. As we have seen, this was, to many nurses, a powerful combination. It allowed them to directly engage valued, valuable, exclusive, and exciting medical knowledge about the body—and to directly access pieces of science and skilled practice—while eliding the questions of social legitimacy facing women who would be physicians.[6] It enabled them to claim social power and authority vis-à-vis other women and particular communities, even if it left open the question of whether these other women and middle-class communities would recognize such claims.

The most active southern champions of professionalism in nursing practice worked, as did their northern colleagues, from positions of relative power. They were, most often, heads of hospital training schools, members of state licensing boards, field representatives of private or philanthropic health programs, or public health nurses. Some were born and raised in the South, but through the first half of the twentieth century, they mostly trained in large, urban, and segregated hospitals in the North.[7] There, white women trained in white hospitals; African American women, in African American hospitals. Only the most tenuous connections existed between the separate and unequal pathways to nursing practice.

The American Nurses Association had always provided one such connection. The ANA had originally organized in 1897 with alumnae associations of schools who met stringent curricula requirements as constituent members. As historian Ellen Baer has pointed out, since American nursing leaders had no power to control training school standards, they chose instead to control the process through which graduate nurses might claim a professionalized practice.[8] Much like the registered nurse credential, an alumnae group's claim to ANA membership would be a badge of a hospital's prestige and a graduate's status. The most prominent African American alumnae associations made such claims. Those at Provident Hospital in Chicago, Lincoln Hospital in New York City, Freedmen's Hospital in Washington, D.C., and Mercy Hospital in Philadelphia had at least some ANA representation in theory, although not always in practice.

But the ANA had reorganized in 1911 with individual states rather than alumnae groups as the association's members. Some northern states offered at least nominal membership to African American training school graduates from Provident, Lincoln, and Mercy hospitals. But neither the southern states' associations nor the District of Columbia's Graduate Nurse Association (GNA) allowed African American members, irrespective of qualifications. The District of Columbia's refusal presented an organizational problem. Despite constant pressure from the national association, it steadfastly refused to extend membership to the more than qualified graduates of the Freedmen's Hospital Training School— perhaps the most prestigious African American training school in the country and a charter member of the original ANA. In response, the ANA had to create a special membership category solely for Freedmen's alumnae. Yet special memberships created continually "vexing problems" of representation, proportional voting privileges, and resources.[9]

The refusal of the District's GNA to grant membership to Freedmen's Alumnae Association also caused episodes of acute political embarrassment. The ANA had moved quickly onto the international stage through the International Council of Nurses (ICN), an organization it had been instrumental in organizing. The association had been able to ignore issues around race and racial practices in its earlier meetings, but by mid-century this was no longer possible. The ANA had been delighted to host the 1947 ICN meeting—the first since the ravages of World War II. But its delight soon turned to dismay when it realized that many international delegates had been formally invited by the District's GNA to come first to the nation's capital on their way to the conference site in Atlantic City, New Jersey. What Gunnar Myrdal had described in his widely read book as a quintessentially American "dilemma" would be on view to the world. The ICN delegates would see how white nurses preached the "American creed" of liberty, justice, and fair treatment even as they denied it to their African Americans colleagues.

"The ICN stands for democracy, tolerance, and freedom of opportunity for all nurses," Josephine Pitman Prescott, one of the conference organizers, wrote to Asby Taylor, the president of the GNA. Prescott, the director of the federal Bureau of Public Health Nursing headquartered in Washington, D.C., both lectured to and pleaded with Taylor. "If the GNA discriminates against colored nurses in any way," she warned, "it will discredit the GNA in the nation's capital." But Prescott ended her letter with an appeal. She felt she had to "beg for the sake of our profession" to make sure that African American nurses were invited to all planned GNA activities.[10] Taylor responded, "surprised" that Prescott might think any discrimination would be shown. Nothing was open to the public. The GNA had retreated behind closed doors of social custom that, in its view, allowed it to do as it wished. The prerogatives of place trumped those of professional representation. The GNA functions, Taylor responded, were private affairs specifically limited to the ICN delegates, "special guests," and its white members.[11]

Mabel Staupers had long been disappointed that the ANA refused to more actively intervene in challenging the discrimination shown to African American nurses by the GNA in particular, and the southern state associations in general.[12] The ANA's official position had been that it was "obliged to accept state nurses associations' decisions."[13] But the fact that the southern states maintained an unassailable color line was, most often, not particularly problematic to the ANA's white nursing leadership. Well into the 1930s, few southern white training schools and even fewer African American ones had the depth and breadth of educational experiences that met national membership criteria. The ostensible issue was not color but criteria—that the politics of race, region, and rural life had left the South with too few women with high school backgrounds applying to too few schools that could provide anything resembling a well-rounded nursing education.

Indeed, both white and African American southern nursing leaders agreed with their national colleagues on many of the issues that seemed problematic in their region. There were, they believed, too many white and African American physicians who owned small, private hospitals subsidized by the day-to-day work of putative students, who only gained medical and surgical experiences and missed those in obstetrics, pediatrics, and nutrition believed necessary for truly professional practice. These women were proud of the contributions they and their students made to the care of patients in these hospitals, but they recognized that some of their responsibilities would not pass muster in larger urban training schools. One such white North Carolinian nursing director reported doing the teaching and the clinical supervision of students—as well as maintaining the hospital's bookkeeping and procurement systems. Another reported that her daily responsibilities ranged from stoking the hospital's boiler, to giving anesthetics, to doing laundry, to assisting at surgery. Yet another told of a friend with a sense of humor about her work. The only thing that this director of nursing had never done, it seemed, was milk cows—but that was only because the hospital had not yet thought to add a dairy.[14]

Moreover, even larger training schools, they agreed, paid little attention to the skills and techniques needed to deal with the "climate conditions" and public health needs of the South. Both white and African American nursing leaders worried about the South's lack of educational opportunities that would prepare nurses for careers in administration and public health.[15] And they shared the same sense of how to address nursing's pressing problems: both linked their regional ambitions for nursing to that of their nation and their national organizations.

African American nursing leaders, of course, had long recognized that the ANA neither would nor could work with them, even if it did allow some official membership. These nurses had formed their own national association, the National Association of Colored Graduate Nurses (NACGN), in 1908. The NACGN and the ANA both fought their own separate battles for the right to set entrance standards for training schools, to control the content of educational curricula for students once admitted to such schools, to legally define and enforce the parameters of professional practice, to stay abreast of changes in health care knowledge and practice, and to create an independent and assertive voice for their particular experience of nursing. They both encouraged the creation of state associations to maintain lines of communication, to keep abreast of changing practices, to create social networks, and, just as importantly, to socialize. But the NACGN had one additional goal: it would work steadfastly to break down the walls of discrimination in nursing.

The North Carolina State Nurses Association

The North Carolina State Nurses Association (NCSNA) was founded in 1902, and like most state nursing associations, it claimed to represent all nurses in the state. But in fact, and in ways that mirrored the national organization, the NCSNA actually represented only a small proportion of white North Carolina nurses. These women had worked hard to access better pre-training education than that available to most North Carolina women. They had attended what were acknowledged to be the better training schools, and they had passed what, by 1931, was the mandatory examination for state registration—and the mandatory credential for the more prestigious and more stable positions in public health, military service, training schools, or hospital administration.[16] The NCSNA, like the ANA, represented an enduring belief about who nurses should be rather than who nurses actually were. And like the ANA, it was self-consciously exclusionary. It was, like all state nursing organizations, the most direct means through which nurses could decide who could enter the more rarified world of professional practice.

This rarified world also positioned itself on the more liberal side of North Carolina politics, reform, and race relations. Although it bridled at one club woman's reference to its place as the "little sisters,"[17] the NCSNA self-consciously linked its professional agenda with that of the moderate, middle-class, white women in North Carolina's Women's Legislative Council, League of Women Voters, and the Federation of Women's Clubs. The NCSNA members, like white club women, were motivated by a genuine belief in reform and an equally genuine need to reinforce racial hierarchies in the rising "New South" of increasing urbanization, commercialized tobacco production, and labor activism.

The NCSNA saw its similarities to white and middle-class associations as another way to challenge class and race stereotypes. It joined such clubwomen in support of prison reform for elderly inmates, federally funded maternal child initiatives, and progressively longer school terms for children that were linked to new child labor laws. It championed tuberculosis prevention campaigns and although separate, at the very least, some institutions for African American men, women, and children. Furthermore, like similar organizations of white club women, the NCSNA coupled the language of moral superiority with acts of what they believed to be a progressive position of moral responsibility. It endorsed, for example, the idea of a home for delinquent African American girls like that already available for white girls. Such a home, the association pointed out, was both a way of supporting African American mothers and "a sign of growing morality in the race."[18] Similarly, it supported the aspirations of African American nurses—insofar as their agenda for the profession would provide more and better-educated nurses from and for separate race communities. From the NCSNA's perspective, the relentless pursuit of better education and higher standards for all nurses worked. While the percentages of white nurses passing the state's registration exam hovered around 70 percent, that of African American nurses rose from 35 percent in 1936 to 50 percent in 1940.[19] Its wish for a separate and equal policy seemed within reach.

But the NCSNA's whole idea of professionalism and professional practice was constantly under assault both from the persistence of untrained (or poorly trained) white and African American nurses and from what the NCSNA explicitly described as the "prejudice" of southern mothers when considering their daughters' educational opportunities.[20] The language of discrimination, in fact, pervaded stories told by white nurses about white nursing in North Carolina. This sense of discrimination was not, in these nurses' minds, about gender per se. Who they were as women remained disconnected from what they were as professionals. Rubye Bowles Bryson, a white public health nurse, claimed, "I never felt discriminated against because I was a woman." Gender was not absent; instead, it was seen as something within their power to control. "I just assumed, no, I'm not discriminated against," Bryson continued, "and by that pure assumption, I wasn't." Stories about discrimination did involve professional representation. In particular, they involved other people's persistent refusal to see nurses as they saw themselves. "The only time I felt discriminated against," Bryson concluded, "was because of the profession I represented."[21]

A certain militancy was taking shape. Shirley Titus had her own story with her own evocative language. States, she pointed out to her colleagues in the ANA's Southern Division in 1935, were increasingly recognizing the importance of more education for nurses. They were beginning to establish and support programs in the institutions they controlled. But some states were pushing nursing education down what she called a "devious and little traversed pathway" of vocational education by encouraging (and paying for) programs in technical schools instead of rooting professional education in the more prestigious liberal arts colleges and universities. Still other states, she argued, were establishing summer institutes for public health nurses—experiences, she sneered, that were "nothing more than one-night stands." Titus was speaking with expertise and from her position as the first professor of nursing education at Vanderbilt University in Nashville, Tennessee. She had been charged by both the university and the Rockefeller Foundation with developing the Vanderbilt University Hospital's traditional three-year training program for nurses into a formal four-year baccalaureate program. She was well on her way to doing so, and as she spoke before the Southern Division, her school of nursing had just welcomed the first class who would graduate with a bachelor's degree in nursing.[22] Her story, then, was one shared in confidence by an accomplished leader among good friends. Gendered dynamics were much more present in Titus's story than in Bryson's. And they were explicitly sexualized. Male educators were more than willing to whisper sweet nothings to unsuspecting nurses, she told her audience, and then leave them broken-hearted in the morning.

But Titus's story was not just about sexualized dynamics. It was also about the relationships of knowledge and power that underpinned such dynamics. It was about insider knowledge that outsiders needed. Nurses, she pointed out, needed to know the "rules of the game" that must be played for any academic program to achieve legitimacy and recognition by educators. And the rules by which educators lived included a firm collegiate base. The half-hearted compromises that existed in nursing were unacceptable. She conjured up the most devious and dispossessed image she could imagine and likened it to nursing. "If nursing education cannot go in the front door of a university as a recognized member," she concluded, it should not demean itself by acting like a thief in the night. It should not attempt to "break in" to higher education "by climbing in the pantry window or by coming up the dumb waiter."[23]

The NCSNA shared with the ANA and other leaders an almost unshakable confidence that such educational opportunities would serve as a defense against nursing's class and race stereotypes; they would be the key that would finally allow others to see them as they saw themselves.[24] The NCSNA was equally unshakable in its belief that these problems cut across race: that both white and African American nurses needed support for what they believed to be their separate and equal agenda of higher standards and better education.[25] Perhaps, Estelle Massey Riddle, the recently elected president of the NACGN, granted, when she spoke immediately after Titus at the same Southern Division meeting. Certainly nursing—and indeed America—needed to work toward a time when the recognition of "RACIAL SIMILARITIES" in issues affecting health and illness became more important than that of "RACIAL DIFFERENCES."[26] But that time had not yet come. There was still, she told her white colleagues, an undeniable "racial relationship to professional opportunity." There were at least opportunities, Riddle pointed out, for southern white nurses to break loose of the traditions, attitudes, and structural inequities that constrained perceptions and practice. There were no opportunities for southern black nurses, no matter how ambitious.

Riddle told this same audience another story. Her story was one shared in hope among well-meaning friends, yet one carefully constructed for southern white ears. And it was a gentle one for such an audience to hear. Her story was not about the inequities that individual white men and women forced upon African Americans. It was, instead, about the more impersonal "King Cotton," and about how "the same group he first enslaved he now forces to the wall with economic insecurity." It was not about entrenched racism. It was instead about a process of economic greed—a greed that "so fixed a stigma on the Negro race in America" and that created a culture that kept the "majority of the negros still gripped if not still enslaved" in poverty and in the isolation of the "complete disinterestedness" of most of America.[27]

Riddle's story was not about southerners. It was about the South. It was about the region's disparities in expenditures for education and about the diseases that knew no color line even as they disproportionately killed African Americans. Her story was not about integration or desegregation, although that was on the NACGN's national agenda. Rather, it was about "realistic" race relations that, for the time being, acknowledged a separate and equal agenda. But another kind of militancy was also taking shape. Nursing's fundamental problems did not cut across race. They were *about* race. "We, as Negro Nurses," she reminded her audience, "no longer wonder if we have a place in the program for the improvement of health in this country." Riddle kept to herself any thoughts she had about the fact that the only place for African American nurses at this Southern Division meeting was in the choir that provided entertainment. But her story ended with a gentle warning. She used the evocative words of the African American poet James Weldon Johnson—words that also underscored African American intellectual traditions. He had advised those who loved their "fair Southland" that if they continued to cling to the vestiges of "an idle age and a musty page," they would soon be left behind in the great march of progress. Nurses, Riddle implied, might be similarly be left behind in a stagnating place cut off from new configurations of professionalism and professional identity.[28]

The State Association of Negro Registered Nurses

The State Association of Negro Registered Nurses (SANRN), founded in 1921 as a state chapter of the NACGN, shared both Riddle's commitment to "realistic" race relations and the ANA's commitment to education, professional standards, and professional practice. Like the NCSNA, it represented only a small proportion of North Carolina's African American nurses and restricted membership to those who met the state's educational criteria for registered nursing practice. This was, as the minutes of the 1923 meeting noted, a more "controversial" and contested decision—and one that reflected at least some members' incorporation of white norms into their own professional sense of self. Several of the most involved and invested African American members of the SANRN, including those who were its founders, had graduated from small and specialized African American training schools that could not meet state standards. These women had to resign until Maye Irwin, visiting from the Freedmen's Hospital, gently pointed out the "injustice" done to older nurses with an overly rigorous interpretations of standards. The struggle continued though. The leadership of SANRN was determined to match the membership criteria of the white NCSNA. In 1925, the association decided "once and for all" that members who graduated between 1912 and 1920 needed only to document two years of training in hospitals of more than twenty-five beds. But any member who had graduated after 1920 had to meet NCSNA and ANA standards. Her education had to have been in a hospital training school with a three-year curriculum and more than fifty beds.[29]

Like the NCSNA, the SANRN reflected a belief about what nurses should be rather than who nurses actually were. But this commitment cost the SANRN more dearly than it did the NCSNA. The SANRN struggled through the 1920s with between fifteen and twenty "faithful" members and some real doubts about whether the organization could even survive.[30] Membership grew slowly through the 1930s, corresponding almost directly with the slowly increasing employment opportunities within North Carolina's African American hospitals and public health system.

The SANRN also positioned itself on the more liberal side of North Carolina politics, reform, and race relations. But it linked its agenda with African American professionals, predominantly male physicians, ministers, and social workers. It endorsed, for example, the privately funded programs of African American social service projects throughout rural North Carolina counties that were organized in the 1920s. Many of these programs had been organized by social worker Lieutenant Lawrence Oxley and supported through the 1930s by donations from African American churches and fraternal organizations.[31] Oxley worked closely with the SANRN around these projects, and in 1930 the association honored his constant collaboration by bestowing upon him the title "male nurse."

SANRN records were much quieter about links to the work of other African American women.[32] It certainly supported the African American women's self-help health initiatives.[33] It replicated the features of many of them. The SANRN's presidential addresses, for example, were often given in churches and were always open to the interested public. Furthermore, individual members depended on these women as "volunteers" who appeared in the SANRN records as helping bring families to their county well-baby and inoculation clinics. It is likely that the North Carolinian African American middle class remained as distant in their support of nursing's work and worth as did that in Georgia. Moreover, any class tensions inherent in the differences between unpaid volunteers and salaried workers, however professional, remained muted in the SANRN's records. But the challenges of class were threaded through these women's lives. Mary Bond Henderson, for example, worked long hours as a nurse in North Carolina's Vance County, first to put her brother through medical school and then as his office nurse when he entered practice. It was their combined work that allowed his family to experience that situation which middle-class and medical white families could take for granted. His wife did not have to work. She could, instead, devote her time to her home and children.[34]

The issue of race was never muted in the SANRN records. At times, its members told stories of possibilities—but possibilities that still acknowledged the tenuousness of its members' place within a segregated system and their struggles to sort through the place of race in their idea of professionalism. Their NCSNA colleagues could assume that their idea of professionalism transcended race—that it involved educational standards, representations, and credentials that existed independent of race. SANRN members never made this same assumption. At the 1930 Annual Meeting, for example, one member told of her loyal white patient who was refused admission to a white hospital by white nurses. The story initially centered on the fact that this refusal was "because of her nurse." But at some point the implications of "because of her nurse" came to this meeting's attention. The phrase implied the possibility that perhaps this African American woman's right to identify herself as a nurse was what the white nurses challenged. The word *nurse* was struck through, and "because of race" inserted in its place.[35]

The SANRN self-consciously saw itself as part of the "rising tide of color." It acknowledged, as another speaker reminded members in 1923, that white supremacy held the key that unlocked the gates of power. The SANRN records never mentioned any alliances with other organizations committed to desegregation. But the organization's members took heart in the belief that they were pushing at the gates and playing some small part in the process of African Americans seizing control of their own institutions.[36]

The SANRN had a clear and persistent sense of what this control meant for its ideas of professionalism and professional practice. In addition to education and professional standards, it meant representation on state nursing governing boards. It also meant equitable employment in public health nursing positions. However progressive North Carolina may have been, the African American nurses hired by the state experienced conditions similar to those in Georgia. They faced restricted employment opportunities, salary differentials, and no possibility of promotion.[37] One nurse, in fact, recalled the promotion to a supervisory position of a young white nurse whom she had trained. "I knew if I'd been white, I'd have been the supervisor," she remembered, "but that job went to her."[38]

But if their white colleagues in the NCSNA had to deal with the constant assaults to the association's ideas of professionalism and professional practice, the SANRN had to deal with something even harder to manage. It met the utter indifference of, and its almost complete invisibility to, the wider white world. With little money and membership, it had to depend on moral suasion. It constantly wrote letters to the Board of Nursing Education, to county public health departments, and to the State Board of Health that invariably went unanswered. By the late

1930s, the SANRN membership was again slowly increasing, but the association itself was demoralized and deteriorating. Members were miserable. They questioned the need to train African American nurses. They focused on the almost overwhelming disadvantages facing African American nurses in the South. And they blamed what they saw as an inefficient organizational structure and what they believed to be problematic qualities of the association's clearly embattled leadership.

Elizabeth McMillan Thompson, the newly elected SANRN president, declared the infighting "embarrassing."[39] In her 1937 presidential address, she laid the issue out clearly. "We have too many people on the outside to fight," she reminded the membership, "instead of fighting ourselves." But it did not help morale when, later on, the SANRN duly noted the ANA's new 1939 resolution that all African American nurses be addressed as "Miss" or "Nurse." It only emphasized a sense of a certain tone-deafness on the part of the ANA to the real issues of southern African American nurses. This resolution may have helped Georgia's African American nurses resist the practice of calling them by their first name only. But the ANA's official institutionalization of the possibility of alternative titles for white and African American nurses legitimated racial hierarchies of practice that had long been reinforced by southern Jim Crow conventions.

Integration Stories

The 1939 resolution did reflect an increasing willingness of the ANA to at least re-engage the issues surrounding the place of African American nurses in its organizational life. Edna Lewis, North Carolina's representative to the ANA's Board of Directors through the early 1940s, reported to the NCSNA that, among other items (such as the ANA's role in planning for the national defense), the board was also reopening issues of membership. It was discussing the possibility of a special section for men who were nurses—a group that had historically been excluded from membership. Furthermore, it had been considering the question of "permitting" African American nurses to join the ANA as individual members. At issue was the question of using the Freedmen's Hospital model as a way of increasing African American membership from the southern states.

Not surprisingly, the NCSNA officially reported back to the ANA that this proposal was "not advisable." It would create an administrative nightmare, and it would complicate "social customs."[40] And not just in the South, the NCSNA argued. It would do so in the North and West, as well. As southern nurses were quick to point out and as northern nurses acknowledged in their surveys, African American nurses did have more practice opportunities outside the South. But these too were largely limited to members of their own communities of color and only if there were enough patients within such communities to justify a full-time African American nursing position.

At the same time, the National Association of Colored Graduate Nurses' policy of "realistic" race relations changed. The integration battle was now clearly on the table. As Elizabeth Jones, the NACGN's national field secretary, told North Carolina's State Association of Negro Registered Nurses in her 1943 visit, the goal now was to "streamline" the national association "so that one day we will just be nurses instead of race groups." More pragmatically and strategically, the NACGN had three specific objectives: it wanted to increase the pressure on the ANA by connecting smaller state associations like North Carolina's SANRN more closely to the NACGN's broader national agenda; it wanted state associations to increase membership numbers by actively recruiting African American nurses who met the ANA's membership criteria; and it wanted to draw more and more powerful white supporters into the fold.

In North Carolina, that meant the Duke Foundation. Established in 1924 by the tobacco, textile, and energy rich Duke family, the foundation supported colleges, hospitals, children's homes, and the state's Methodist Church. Jones peppered the SANRN with questions about their relationship to the foundation. Did the Duke Foundation, a longtime supporter of African American hospitals, know what African American nurses were doing in the state? How was the SANRN going to get the foundation-supported hospital at Duke University to hire African American nurses? Where were the other lay supporters of the SANRN's agenda—and why weren't they members?[41] The SANRN had no interest in pursuing a relationship with the Duke Foundation, but it was willing to test the nursing waters. It sent a letter to the white North Carolina State Nurses Association in 1944 requesting membership. And it received, in return, a copy of that association's by-laws with the notation that only white nurses were accepted. The NCSNA was concerned about integration at that time, but its idea of integration involved creating new state Board of Nursing Education standards that would integrate public health nursing content into training school curricula.[42]

Nationally, the pressure to integrate nursing was increasing. Not coincidentally, the National League for Nursing Education (NLNE), which was the first professional association formed by nurses and was responsible for setting the national educational standards that were so close to the heart of the project of professionalizing nursing, abruptly changed its membership policies. There had always been close ties between the ANA and the NLNE. The NLNE required ANA membership for admission. This requirement, of course, had precluded the organizational participation of southern African American nursing educators. But by 1942, the NLNE had grown tired of waiting for the ANA to address the issue of desegregation. Unwilling to deal with both the idea and the administration of different categories for different members, the NLNE simply rewrote its by-laws. It borrowed them from the National Organization for Public Health Nursing, which had always been integrated, and made constituent members individuals rather than states. The ANA (and its state associations like the NCSNA) were immediately isolated as the only nursing associations that deliberately refused to admit qualified African American nurses as members as a matter of right.

For many in the ANA, this continued resistance was morally indefensible; for others, it may have become politically indefensible. The no longer unthinkable plan of individual African American membership would create a disproportionately powerful group of African American nurses outside of state control. In 1946, the president of the NCSNA was finally able to report on her attendance at a "history making" national convention. The ANA platform endorsed better hours and living conditions for nurses, collective bargaining, and the removal of barriers to full employment and the professional development of nurses from minority groups "as rapidly as possible." The NCSNA president noted that this latter plank was no longer wishful thinking or the personal agenda of the association's more liberal leadership. It and the concomitant decision to allow individual African American membership had been endorsed by a "large majority" of the delegates, who represented nurses from all states all across the country. Perhaps, she suggested, it was time for the NCSNA to recognize that this issue would not go away. "The Florida Nurses Association has found a way to admit Negro nurses," she told her members. In 1942 its strategy had been to simply eliminate "white" from its by-laws and hope no African American nurses appeared where they were not wanted. "It may be well," she concluded, "for North Carolina to study their plan."[43]

But in 1946, the NCSNA also faced what it saw as a more immediate assault to its ideas of professionalism and professional practice. The recently appointed North Carolina Medical Care Commission, after surveying the postwar health care needs of the state, had painted a grim picture.[44] Of all 48 states, the NCSNA president reported, North Carolina was 47th in military service rejections; 45th in numbers of physicians per population; 41st in numbers of hospital beds; and 38th in infant mortality.[45] The solution, all recognized, was to be hospitals. In 1946, the nation embarked on a massive hospital building program financed through the federal Hospital Survey and Construction Act, also known as the Hill-Burton Act in honor of its sponsors. But to staff those new hospitals, both the North Carolina Hospital Association and the Medical Society of North Carolina proposed rewriting the Nurse Practice Act, long the heart of what nursing saw as its control over professional practice. Both the Hospital Association and the Medical Society, like their affiliated organizations across the country, wanted a new category of nursing personnel, the licensed practical nurse (LPN), to meet anticipated staffing shortages.

Like other nursing organizations across the country, the NCSNA opposed such a move. North Carolina, it argued, needed better-educated white and African American nurses. It did not need more poorly trained practitioners who might compromise patient care. And, given projected salary scales that suggested LPNs would "barely make a living wage," it certainly did not need poorer women entering nursing who would replay the class and race associations they had struggled to escape.[46] No nursing organization—northern or southern—successfully opposed the LPN movement. The combination of postwar America's acute nursing shortages and dramatically rising demands by hospitals made the movement appear almost inevitable. But the NCSNA, unlike most northern nursing organizations, believed it could not even risk the appearance of opposition. It faced the limits of its particular idea of professionalism. Avoiding engaging with the social legitimacy of women's claims to formal medical knowledge may have worked in an earlier era, but now it left North Carolina nurses particularly vulnerable to direct engagement with the powerful world of white male privilege. The NCSNA felt that it had no public support—or even acknowledgment—and experienced a sense of indifference and invisibility similar to that which the SANRN had long known. Thus it felt "compelled to cooperate" with an initiative it opposed "rather than submit the nursing profession of North Carolina to the public view as being antagonistic to the Medical Society and the Hospital Association."[47] A new Nurse Practice Act received legislative approval in 1947.

At the same time that the NCSNA was capitulating on one issue, it was slowly moving ahead of the North Carolina Medical Society on another: race relations. By 1947, the NCSNA had quietly removed "white" from its own by-laws. It had no choice because it had to comply with federal regulations if the association were to represent nurses as a collective bargaining unit. It did want to, particularly at the much-anticipated 600-bed hospital that the state was planning at the University of North Carolina in Chapel Hill—a hospital that would also come with new opportunities for nursing education and practice. But the NCSNA also recognized its increasing isolation from the professional world of the ANA, from its own progressive traditions, and from those of influential white club women now participating in the state's interracial Hill-Burton commissions that were recommending how many dollars would go to which (still-segregated) hospitals.[48] While the North Carolina Medical Society stood firm on segregation, the question among the NCSNA leadership was no longer *if* African Americans should be admitted as members. The question now was how that would happen.

The SANRN paid these particular policies and politics no mind. It had long worried about untrained nurses, especially white practical nursing, and the threat this presented to its own ideas about professional nursing practice. But it had also long abandoned any plans to directly engage that issue. Its annual meetings also brought little information to its members about collective bargaining or employment opportunities. African American nurses were and would be employed by affected hospitals to care for patients in segregated wards, but they knew their numbers would to be too small to have a substantive impact on deliberations. The association had turned its attention to much more treacherous politics. The SANRN also knew that the desegregation question was no longer if but how. Tentative contact between the SANRN and the NCSNA had begun in 1944, and negotiations began in earnest in 1947. The sides remained far apart. Even language remained problematic. The SANRN believed the goal to be a merger of the two associations, while the NCSNA thought the goal to be how to incorporate African Americans into a white organization.[49]

Elizabeth McMillan Thompson was the SANRN's most prominent voice in these negotiations.[50] Thompson represented all that nurses should be, irrespective of race. She was the North Carolina–born daughter of what she described as "educated and influential" parents. Her father was a physician, and her mother, who once served in church missions in Africa and Florida, worked to make sure all the children in their community knew how to read and write.[51] Thompson had spent two years at the African American Shaw University in Raleigh before graduating from the Freedmen's Hospital Training School for Nurses in 1928. She had earned additional public health nursing credentials at Howard University in Washington, D.C. Committed to nursing's professionalism agenda, she was, as a Freedmen's alumna, a career-long member of the American Nurses Association; the National League for Nursing Education; the State Association of Negro Registered Nurses, whose presidency she held in 1936; and the National Association of Colored Graduate Nurses, whose presidency she held in 1942.[52]

Thompson also represented all that African American nurses should be. She took pride in thinking of herself as North Carolina's first black public health nurse and in the work she did with her rural Cumberland County community during the smallpox epidemic that had drawn her back to her home state. She remained in public health nursing for thirty-five years, supervising midwives, organizing TB identification and prevention programs, and running the well-baby, venereal disease, and inoculation clinics. As an African American, she experienced the salary inequities, the contradictions, and the tenuousness of her place in a white health care system. When the Board of Health cut her salary from $37.50 to $25 in 1932, she considered resigning and returning to her parents' home.[53] But Thompson also had the race consciousness to recognize that in all probability a white nurse would be appointed to fill her position. She stayed in the position, knowing she could not support herself with such a meager salary, and had to assume a second position as the nurse for the nearby Fayetteville State College in exchange for free room and board.

Thompson was remarkably sanguine about race and race relations. "I knew the situation in North Carolina before I went off to nursing school," she later remembered, "so I just sort of took it in stride." But she also saw herself as fiercely protective of her individual rights. "I didn't take any foolishness," she asserted, "and there were only certain things they could say to me." Her recollections were of supportive relationships with white professionals—be they physicians or teachers. In fact, she once found herself teaching white nursing students. "Can you imagine that," she wondered, "in the days of segregation?"[54]

But the negotiations over membership did take place in the days of segregation, and the most important issue—in fact, the only issue on the table—involved the social place of African American nurses in the NCSNA, a minefield through which all participants trod carefully. As the SANRN had noted in a special 1947 executive session, the exact wording of the ANA's 1946 position meant that it would accept individual African American members only *after* they had been refused membership in their state association. But in March of 1947, the NCSNA asked the SANRN to delay its formal application until after all the details about membership were resolved. At issue, of course, was the critical and explicit question: Would African American nurses be willing, if members, to conform to "southern social customs" that enforced segregation? Would they be willing to abide by local hotel and restaurant regulations that prohibited service to African Americans? Would they conform to established seating arrangements in local assembly halls and other organizational venues that placed them in the back of the room? The SANRN agreed to delay their formal application, and, after a year of what the NCSNA, at least, described as "free and open discussions," the SANRN did agree to respect such customs. The recognition of their rightful place as professionals mattered more.

But at the same time that the SANRN was capitulating on one issue, it was also creating opportunities around another. It saw itself as using the important fact of membership to prepare for incremental challenges to the rules of white privilege. They were probably well aware of the work of their African American nursing colleagues in Florida. These women had also agreed to respect southern segregated social customs and then proceeded to test them at every opportunity. Prohibitions against integrated dining and socializing remained inviolable. But as Mary Elizabeth Carnegie remembered, those against integrated seating arrangements in meetings were more pliable. Carnegie, a Rosenwald Foundation scholar, the architect of Florida's desegregation strategy, and soon to emerge as a national nursing leader, told of a plan in which she and her colleagues would arrive early to their state association meetings and deliberately seat themselves in chairs scattered throughout the room. White colleagues arriving later had a choice. They could maintain segregated seating and stand throughout the entire meeting, or they could sit in an integrated space. White nurses eventually chose to sit. These kinds of stories suggested to the SANRN that it had room for maneuvering around the politics of power. And it maintained the language it chose to represent its goals. In June of 1948, the issue of what the NCSNA presented as "membership applications" by African American nurses and what the SANRN presented as a "merger" between two associations went before their respective members.[55]

By 1948 most NCSNA members, reassured that segregated social customs were not to be threatened, supported African American membership. But that year's annual meeting still needed to provide a carefully orchestrated space where resistance could be recognized, recorded, sometimes rebutted, but always reassured. The minutes of the 1948 meeting when this issue reached the floor went on for pages, and, in one of the few instances in the organization's history, they recorded the names of every participant in the question-and-answer session. Why can't African American nurses accept the ANA's offer of individual membership? The tide is turning. Where North Carolina was once one of eleven southern states not accepting such membership, it is now one of only nine. Mississippi, another member pointed out, had been accepting African American members since 1947. "Now we in North Carolina and pretty much over the nation," she admitted, "think of Mississippi as the deepest of the Deep South." She only spoke partly in jest when she called to NCSNA members' pride in their sense of themselves as progressive. "We can't allow Mississippi," she reminded them, "to get ahead of North Carolina."[56]

But what if the NCSNA can't find desegregated venues? The North Carolina Board of Education has been finding desegregated venues since the early 1940s for nurses taking registration exams—including some in the best hotels in Raleigh. What about the "ruin of the social life of the organization"? African American nurses are seeking only "educational advantages." Their concern, in fact, is that they will have to forgo their own social life, and they actually need assurances from us that they can continue to have their own separate social activities.[57] And what about the most important question? What if we are jeopardizing "our position as the superior dominant race"? Well, first there is the pragmatic issue of sheer numbers. There are 256 African American members of the SANRN and 3,000 white members of the NCSNA. And then there is the issues of dues. Their dues are $3.00, and ours are $13. In reality, one member pointed out, "I don't think we are going to be overcome with them as members."[58] But as the president of the NCSNA pointed out, an equally significant issue was class. SANRN members were "educated Negroes," and as such, they promised to be "very sensible" about social customs.[59] The NCSNA president admitted that the SANRN leaders had refused to put this in writing. Still, she continued, we can be assured, because "it is not the educated Negro that causes trouble in this respect. If you ride on a bus in the South, the educated Negro in there will not insist on sitting on the front seat; it is the other type, and I think you are going to be dealing with this higher type of Negro."[60]

The SANRN's annual meeting just a few weeks later was, by contrast, presented in its records as one of almost total silence. It noted the unanimous passage of a "merger agreement" that spoke of abiding by "southern customs" and of a discussion of the ways in which this phrase was to be "literally defined."[61] Its meeting in November of 1948 to finalize its letter of application to the NCSNA acknowledged the presence of some opposition within the SANRN, although its records remained silent about whether this was to the merger itself or to the terms that made the merger possible. Of more importance was the recognition of the "progressive step" that was about to be taken. This would not be a blind step. "We realize," the SANRN wrote in its application letter to the NCSNA, "that there may be a few difficulties in such matters as meeting places where social customs are rigidly observed." But it also characterized such differences as "minor" and looked forward to a future in which white and

African American women "will approach such difficulties as professional women."[62] When the SANRN dissolved itself voluntarily on June 25, 1949, it issued a press release: "Nurses Make Historic Decision."[63]

The Meaning of Integration

On one level, the story of the integration of the NCSNA might be told in a fairly straightforward manner. It presented no immediate threat to white supremacy and the Jim Crow laws that supported it. The integration model established after negotiations between the SANRN and the NCSNA included the high $13 NCSNA dues to impede black membership and a new organizational structure that planned educational presentations in desegregated venues but social gatherings in those that prohibited African American clients. The SANRN offered no sustained challenge to this model. It focused instead on the importance of nurses as leaders in what they acknowledged would be incremental assaults on white supremacy. SANRN leaders may have chafed at the subordination of their place to that of their white nursing peers within an only ostensibly desegregated NCSNA. But these women looked not only to their state nursing world. They also looked to the wider world of African American professional practice. They could now claim their place as "first" among the physicians, social workers, and ministers with whom they worked.

But the stories surrounding the integration of the NCSNA also suggest more than just the relationships of power between entrenched white privilege and African American agency. Of course, the nature of these relationships was fundamentally different for white and African American nursing leaders. Although both the NCSNA and the SANRN were conscious of persistent discrimination, the NCSNA and its members still had the privilege of being blind to their own racism. One white Halifax County public health nurse, for example, might consider her African American colleague, Edith MacNeil Holmes, a good friend and colleague. This white woman would challenge social customs by inviting Holmes to join her family for Sunday supper. Still, as Holmes recalled, that same nurse could and would reproduce racial hierarchies behind closed doors. "They would always set up a separate little table for me, next to theirs," Holmes remembered, "although there was plenty of room for me to eat at the table with them." Holmes said nothing, "but deep down inside, I really resented it."[64]

Still, stories like Holmes's, and like those told between and among African American and white nurses, did succeed in constructing a particular narrative where nurses might come together at least around an idea of professionalism, if not around the reality of North Carolina's segregated social and nursing practices. These stories, constructed by both white and African American nurses, emphasized a shared professional commitment that muted sustained discussions of race and racism between both groups and highlighted assumptions about class status that might be a bridge across a racial divide. These stories told of a belief in desegregation—not necessarily as an idea in and of itself, but rather as a tool to strengthen these women's political, social, and professional position with regard to the broader world of medicine, the academy, and the country. Moreover, this idea and the stories that supported it may have been more than wishful words. As one sociologist who had studied race relations at the Presbyterian Hospital in Chicago noted in 1960, the status of professional was the African American nurse's strongest weapon against discrimination. If the hospital were to run smoothly, the hospital hierarchy and nursing's occupational place within that hierarchy had to be respected irrespective of the race of the individual nurse. Her African American informants agreed. One African American nurse told a story about how her white nursing supervisor took a white nursing student to task for questioning her order. No matter what the student might feel about the place or the competence of an African American woman, the white supervisor told her student, she still had to respect and obey that individual as a graduate nurse.[65]

These particular stories, though, were fraught with problems. The meaning of words like *desegregation* and *integration, membership* and *merger* was left ambiguous. Thus they assumed different meanings to different individuals in different contexts, and important story lines were left undeveloped. What about the NCSNA's constant vigilance for signs of class discrimination that thwarted the possibility of recognizing the ways in which it perpetuated its own forms of class and race discrimination?[66] And what of the SANRN's willingness to defer outright equality for some measure of acceptance by white nurses? This was a trade-off some African American physicians in other southern places were willing to make; it was one North Carolina's own physicians were not.[67]

The processes around desegregation in North Carolina, not surprisingly, were tenuous and unstable. But the stories about this issue were still critically important to both white and African American nursing leaders. They provided visibility and power not just for nursing in the state of North Carolina but, more importantly, for power and visibility within national communities. A decade later, Marie B. Noell, the executive director of the NCSNA, would recreate a story for the readers of the *American Journal of Nursing* about how North Carolina nurses were still first among equals. Her story was about how, in their desegregation decision, they were always "way ahead" of the communities in which they lived and practiced, and about how they were always cited in the press as an example of how all people could work together.[68] And Estelle Riddle, privately dismayed about the enduring lack of African American representation within the ANA, would speak to the nation's African American community with pride. Other African American leaders were now looking to nursing, she would write in *Crisis,* to find out why and how they "did" it. No other all-Negro organization, she pointed out, had as yet taken the "all important step of dissolving its national body."[69] Thus, desegregation, in North Carolina at least, was neither a sham nor a shining moment. Some small but significant steps toward desegregation were achieved and maintained. But these were not done by giving voice to stories or by sharing experiences and aspirations. Desegregation was achieved through deliberate silences. "I could tell you stories," an African American nurse told her interviewer in 1970, "but I won't." And her interviewer, a fellow nurse, did not ask why not.[70]

CHAPTER 7

Who Is a Nurse?

I N 2003, THE YALE UNIVERSITY FRIENDS, colleagues, and former
students of John Devereaux Thompson created *Compelled by Data* to
memorialize the life and work of a giant in his field. He was remembered
as "a man of many parts"—a nurse, health care administrator, student
of the history of hospital architecture, health services researcher, educator, and mentor.[1] Thompson and his colleague Robert Fetter had developed the system of Diagnosis Related Groups (DRGs) as a way to
statistically analyze and ultimately improve the problematic variations of quality care and costs within clinically coherent disease categories. The federal government, seeking to contain the escalating costs
of Medicare, its health insurance program for elders, appropriated DRGs
as the basis of its new Prospective Payment System, and other insurers
quickly followed.[2]

The conversion of DRGs from Thompson and Fetter's clinically
grounded research tool that allowed comparisons among hospitals into
a new kind of payment system transformed the nation's system of health
care reimbursement in the early 1980s. Now used to link particular clus-
ters of diseases or treatments to a fixed payment, it substantively changed
the hospital experience for both patients and staff. To survive in a new
fixed-rate system that allowed hospitals to keep what they did not spend,
patients were admitted later in their illness experience and discharged
sooner to an expanding system of outpatient facilities. It was a demanding if not traumatic transition for all. Thompson, his friends remembered, had joked that his trademark vest had become a "flak jacket"
against the barbs of hospital administrators.[3]

Thompson's friends, colleagues, and former students wrote of his
overarching concern for the welfare of patients within the institution he
loved to study and improve. They all connected that concern with his

experiences as a nurse. Thompson, like many young men and women who entered nurses training, had wanted to attend college. But an unexpected illness had derailed these plans. As his former student and fellow nurse Edward Halloran recounted, Thompson's mother encouraged nursing school. He would have free room and board and, upon graduation, a marketable skill that he could use to put himself through college later. In 1937 he entered Bellevue Hospital's Mills School of Nursing for Men in New York City, one of the few training schools for men in the country. After graduation, Thompson served in the navy during World War II. His position was as a pharmacist's mate because the military nurse corps refused to admit men or African American women.

After the war, Thompson returned to New York and earned a degree in business from City College of New York in 1947 while working nights as a nurse on Bellevue's men's prison ward. Thompson had by then decided on a career in hospital administration. On the recommendation of one of his teachers, he went to a new program at Yale University, where he remained for the rest of his professional career. Thompson maintained a strong nursing identity. He held a faculty appointment in Yale's School of Nursing, served on the Board of the Visiting Nurse Association of New Haven, and mentored a new generation of nurse researchers interested in the vexing problem of quantifying the impact of nursing care on patients' experiences. As he looked back on his earlier nursing work, what had once seemed only a fairly secure way to earn a living now appeared entirely different. "What I didn't realize at the time," he told Halloran, "was that that experience would mark me forever."[4]

Thompson's life and work was not typical of the quieter lives led by most American nurses. But his story and his faith in the power of quantitative statistical data allow one to look more closely at the women and some men who chose to do the work of nursing—those who chose to trade work for knowledge. Like those before, this chapter tells stories, but it also draws on census data and educational statistics to chart a broader picture of the intersections of gender, race, and social place among American nurses. As this chapter moves the story of American nursing into the latter half of the twentieth century, it also uses these data, with those in national sample surveys of registered nurses, to argue that the identity and the work of nursing supported the class aspirations and genuine social mobility of diverse groups of women and of some men like John Thompson. Nursing allowed women and men to trade work that transformed the care provided in American homes, hospitals, and health care systems for the knowledge that changed their sense of themselves and their social place. Yet this trade worked more powerfully for some women and men than it did for others.

Gender, Race, and Marital Status in Early Twentieth-Century America

The number of men and women who identified themselves as "professional nurses" exploded in the early decades of the twentieth century (see Appendix, Table A.1). The overwhelming majority of these individuals were white women like Corrine Kern's narrator, Daisy Barnwell Jones, Alice Burrell, Emitt Wimbash, and the women of St. Luke's. But despite the gendered images in the public's imagination, it was not until the 1930s that trained nursing became predominantly women's work. Women represented 91 percent of all such nurses in 1900, and their proportionate representation rose through the succeeding decades until, by 1930, they represented 98 percent of all trained nurses. And despite the racial images, it was not until the 1930s that trained nursing became predominately white women's work. White women represented 89 percent of all women who identified as professional nurses in 1900, and by 1930 they represented 95 percent of all such women (Table A.2).

The dominance of white women as nurses, however, did not come at the expense of African American women. Throughout the early decades of the twentieth century, the proportional representation of African American women who identified as professional nurses remained fairly stable at approximately 3 percent of all nurses. The dominance of white women in the profession came at the expense of men. Men represented 9 percent of those identifying themselves as professional nurses in 1900, but their proportional representation dropped steadily until, by 1930, they represented only 2 percent (Table A.2). As students, men felt the disdain of female nurses for whom gender biases were as strong as racial ones. "There is hardly a day that we are not called orderlies by the charge nurse on the wards," one male student wrote in 1925, "and our work consists mainly of carrying bedpans, urinals and giving rectal treatments, the female nurses do the rest."[5] As graduates, they had no place as colleagues within nursing organizations, and they had few opportunities for postgraduate study.[6]

Yet even as the proportionate number of men identifying as professional nurses was dropping, the racial distribution among them was significantly changing. Through the early twentieth century, professional nursing was steadily becoming the work of white men as well as white women. While white men represented 80 percent of all men identifying as professional nurses in 1900, by the 1920s 98 percent were white (Table A.2). In many respects, this is hardly surprising. African American men were the group with the fewest opportunities to train as nurses. The historical record shows little evidence of a place for them within African American training schools within either African American or white-run hospitals. Nor did they seem to find a place within the psychiatric hospitals where the vast majority of male nurses trained. More surprisingly, African American men were simultaneously losing their place among untrained or practical nursing as well. African American men represented 14 percent of all men who identified themselves as such in 1900. But by 1930, they represented only 1 percent (Table A.3). Practical as well as professional nursing had become the work of white men.

This was in part because all nurses needed some education to read orders and record observations, and professional nurses needed at least some high school education to calculate complicated medication doses, to interpret complex surgical orders, and to summarize and record their patients' changing clinical states. African American men did have fewer educational opportunities than white men, and most had to leave school and join the labor market to support themselves and their families. In 1900, 53 percent of white boys between the ages of 5 and 19 were enrolled in school, but only 30 percent of African American boys were.

But by 1930, increased public educational opportunities drew proportionately more African American boys into school. The 71 percent of white boys enrolled represented a 34 percent increase, but the 60 percent of African American boys in school represented an increase of 106 percent. Moreover, the ratios of white and African American boys enrolled in school in 1930 (71% to 60%) approached that of white and African American girls (71% to 61%).[7] By 1930, that is, the pool of African American men theoretically eligible for admission to nursing school approached that of their white counterparts. Yet their actual numbers in nursing school remained negligible. African American men may well have stayed away from nursing because they felt more vulnerable to its gendered images. They may also have been kept away because black women's hands on white bodies may have raised some anxieties, but those of black men on white bodies created unthinkable sexual images.

Most white and African American women who identified as nurses were single, although white female nurses were significantly more likely to be single than were African American nurses (Table A.4). But through the 1920s, trends began shifting for all white working women as more and more remained in the labor market after marriage, leaving only when expecting their first child.[8] By 1930, the numbers of single white female nurses had dropped to 73 percent, and those married and living with their husbands had risen from 5 percent in 1920 to 12 percent. The numbers of single African American women had similarly dropped to 43 percent by 1930, and those married and living with their husbands also rose from 21 percent in 1920 to 26 percent (Table A.4a).

Still, white female nurses, like other white women in general, remained significantly more likely to leave paid nursing or other forms of work after marriage than were African American female nurses. Married African American nurses, sometimes by choice but more often by racial practices that sharply curtailed the employment options and opportunities of African American men, had to work in paid employment to help support themselves and their families. But these women were also much more vulnerable than white female nurses when separated from their husbands or when they found themselves widowed. Thirty-two percent of these African American female nurses remained in the nursing workforce when separated or widowed, as compared to 14 percent of white female nurses in similar circumstances (Table A.4a). African American female nurses may well have had the same social and emotional supports from families and friends during these trying periods. But it does seem that they were less likely than their white peers to be able to depend upon them for economic assistance (Figure 7.1).

By 1940, however, the patterns of work and marital status of white and African American women identifying as nurses became virtually indistinguishable (Figure 7.2). Sixty-eight percent of white female nurses were single as were 63 percent of African American nurses. Similarly, 18 percent of white married female nurses remained in the workforce as

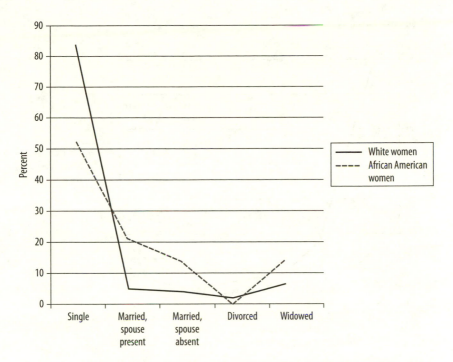

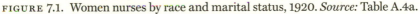

FIGURE 7.1. Women nurses by race and marital status, 1920. *Source:* Table A.4a.

did 21 percent of African American ones (Table A.4a). In addition, more single and married white and African American women identifying as nurses worked than did their counterparts who worked in other kinds of positions: in 1940, 46 percent of single American women worked, and 16 percent of married women did.[9] Both white and African American female nurses were also more educated than their community counterparts and, because of their education, had more employment possibilities open to them either within or outside nursing. By 1940, all American nurses needed at least a high school diploma to enter nursing school. In 1940, only 28 percent of all white women and 8 percent of all African American women had graduated from high school.[10]

But the comparisons mask the devastating effects of the 1930s economic depression on all nurses.[11] Calls for private duty nursing disappeared as fewer and fewer patients could afford the costs of nursing care. The federal Civil Works Administration (CWA) stepped in and provided

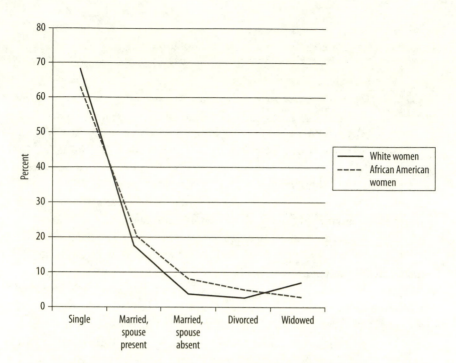

FIGURE 7.2. Women nurses by race and marital status, 1940. *Source:* Table A.4a.

temporary employment in hospitals and on community public health projects for thousands of white nurses and hundreds of African American ones. In Richmond, Virginia, for example, CWA funds supported the salaries of seven white female nurses and three African American female nurses to work in city hospitals, and those of twenty white female nurses and twenty-one African American female nurses to work in its public health programs.[12] Later monies, available through the new Social Security Act, allowed some of these nurses, particularly those who worked for public health care agencies, to assume more permanent positions.

A more stable employment solution came as hospitals, experiencing their own economic pressures, discovered that hiring private duty nurses to work as hospital staff nurses was significantly less expensive than running a formal training program. American nursing leadership had long urged the hiring of graduate staff nurses as a way to relieve students of their complete responsibility for the care of the hospital's patients. But hospitals and the nurses who ran their training schools preferred the stability (and often more easily controlled) student workforce. Preferences began changing in the 1930s. As Jean Whelan argues, hospitals discovered that hiring private duty nurses into temporary staff positions gave them much more financial flexibility. Private duty nurses, unlike students, could be let go when the patient census fell and rehired as soon as it rose.[13] Over 800 hospital-based schools of nursing closed during the 1930s.[14] These were almost exclusively white schools. As Darlene Clark Hine has shown, few white or integrated hospitals sought the services of private duty African American female nurses, and most of the black hospitals seemed content to continue to rely on students' work with their patients.[15] Indeed, between 1930 and 1940, the distribution of marital status and workforce participation patterns of African American female nurses remained stable. But in this same time period, work patterns of married white female nurses began to resemble that of their African American colleagues. By 1930, data on African American female nurses already reflected their tenuous economic place. By 1940, the similar data on white female nurses suggests the extent to which this tenuousness was shared by all nurses (see Figure 7.2).

Worth and Work after the Great Depression

The employment picture dramatically changed again during the 1940s. World War II brought an acute demand for more nurses for both civilian and military service. Nurses who had been desperate for positions now found more than they imagined. After the 1929 stock market crash, Lizzie Gary Bolton's husband, for example, had lost his lifetime savings and his position as Georgia's field secretary at the Southern Baptist Theological Seminary. Bolton, a white North Carolina native, had no choice but to return to work, and with few nursing positions available, she took a commissioned job as a traveling salesperson for the *Farmer's Wife*, a magazine written exclusively for farm women and available only through personal subscription.[16] Bolton put her three children through college selling subscriptions, traveling alone on isolated rural roads with a gun in her car's glove box and the confidence of feeling "perfectly capable," her son remembered, of putting a bullet in the head of any man who attempted to rape or molest her." But the promise of more money and an even more stable work life brought her back to nursing in the early 1940s. She took a series of hospital positions that paid enough to allow her to finally realize her "life long dream" of buying her own home.[17]

The steadily escalating demand also relaxed some racial barriers to practice. Florence Jacob Edmunds, an African American nurse, had turned to sewing to supplement her husband's salary during the 1930s. Edmunds, from Pittsfield, Massachusetts, trained at Lincoln Hospital in New York City after the white school of nursing in her own community had refused to admit her. An extraordinarily talented nurse, she won a scholarship for postgraduate study at Teachers College and worked at the Henry Street Settlement House after receiving her degree. Her husband, another Pittsfield native, followed her to New York City, but they both returned, believing that the small city of Pittsfield was a better place to raise their family. Edmunds wanted and needed to work. But in her mind Pittsfield, with its small African American community, was still not ready to conceive of the idea of an African American nurse. That changed in the 1940s. Edmunds found that Pittsfield was so ready to consider an African American nurse that both the local visiting nurse association and, she ironically noted, the hospital that had once refused her admission to its training school competed for her services.[18] She chose to join the visiting nurse association.[19]

But attempts to draw nurses back into the workforce could not meet demand. For the first time, the federal government had to create a massive program that subsidized both white and African American nurses training through the creation of the Cadet Nurse Corps in 1943. Administered by U.S. Public Health Service, the Cadet Nurse Corps effectively recruited women, paid both their educational and living expenses, expedited their training in schools that met accepted standards, and assigned them to essential civilian and military positions "for the duration of the present war." A remarkably effective program, it ultimately trained over 124,000 white and 3,000 African American nurses.[20] The numbers of nurses rose during this period (Table A.1). But the demand grew even more sharply.

In many respects, this sharply rising demand for nurses in the 1940s and 1950s brought the mutuality of the processes embodied in the practices of medicine and nursing again to the forefront. Nineteenth-century processes were about ideas about science and scientific practice, while those of the twentieth century were about the stunning achievements those ideas and practices had brought about. But the same reciprocal processes that had first played themselves out in the latter half of the nineteenth century—trading scientific knowledge for increasingly responsible and authoritative work—re-emerged in the later twentieth century in hospitals as physicians and nurses sought ways to treat and care for critically ill patients. Physicians yet again needed well-educated and well-trained nurses to accurately observe and record their patients' signs and symptoms, to interpret their meanings, and to act independently to save their patients' lives. Nurses, in turn, needed physicians to share particular medical content that would broaden their knowledge and support their authority, indeed, their responsibility, to act quickly and competently on what they saw.

As Julie Fairman, Joan Lynaugh, and Arlene Keeling have argued, acute shortages of nurses to provide what was increasingly recognized as life-saving treatments to men and women with complicated cardiac, surgical, and medical conditions led physicians and nurses in local and hospital-based settings across the country to again renegotiate the boundaries between medical and nursing knowledge and practice. In newly created critical care units, cardiac care units, and recovery room suites, alliances with supportive physicians allowed talented and ambitious nurses to broaden the scope of their particular practices. They assumed increasing responsibility for procedures and treatments that had once been the sole domain of physicians. And they assumed their own sense of authority and identity as specialist nurses deployed not just in their relationships with physicians but also in their relationships with their fellow nurses.[21]

Their fellow nurses remained in short supply, driven, as in the 1920s and as experienced by the women of St. Luke's in New York City, by the insatiable demands of hospitals for nurses. By 1944, the American Hospital Association had warned that close to 23 percent of American hospitals had closed wards and operating rooms because they had too few nurses.[22] And by 1950 it reported over 22,000 unfilled nursing positions among its member hospitals.[23] These were troubling numbers. The federal and state monies available through the Hill-Burton Act explicitly made the hospital the center of the American health care system. By

1951, the Hill-Burton Act had added 88,000 new hospital beds across the country. By 1968, at the end of its funding, it had financed the building of 9,200 new hospitals, with over 400,000 new beds for patients needing nurses.[24]

Nurses were not only in short supply, but as in the early twentieth century, the prevailing concern among nursing leaders was that many nurses lacked the necessary education and training to meet future demands.[25] There was little new in American nursing leadership's concerns, but as Joan Lynaugh has pointed out, what was new in the latter half of the twentieth century was the political will and public monies to do something about changing the structure of nursing education. In the later twentieth century, Hill-Burton financing and the passage of Medicare made health and hospital care a public as well as a private concern. Investment in the education of nurses able to provide such care followed suit. As President Lyndon Johnson recognized when he signed the federal Nurse Training Act of 1964, "Nurses must perform functions once done by physicians." To this end, the Nurse Training Act poured over 4 billion dollars into basic and advanced nursing education over the next ten years.[26]

The Nurse Training Act helped change both the structure of and opportunities for access to nursing education for tens of thousands of American men and women. And changes in the structure of American higher education had an equally profound effect. In 1960 traditional hospital-based training programs accounted for over 80 percent of all nursing students. Yet by 1970 only 16 percent of all nursing students were enrolled in these programs, and by 1980 almost all such programs had closed their doors. Increasingly stringent accreditation standards and the decisions by private insurance companies to no longer consider the costs of nursing education as an allowable expense to be added to a patient's hospital bill had substantially increased the costs of running such schools. But it was the community college movement that eventually spelled their death knell.[27]

Enter the Community College

Experiences with the Cadet Nurse Corps of World War II showed that nurses could learn the necessary content and understand the characteristic practices of different clinical areas in less time than the three years traditionally allocated in hospital-based diploma programs. To qualify for federal monies and to speed the education of more nurses during wartime, training schools had to redesign curricula from a three-year experience to one that could be completed in thirty months. This redesign, in turn, laid the groundwork for thinking about different kinds of curricular structures. Much as earlier twentieth-century dissatisfaction with opportunities for public health nursing education laid the foundation for baccalaureate programs in nursing, so later twentieth-century dissatisfaction with the ability of traditional programs to train adequate numbers of nurses for hospital-based practice paved the way for another kind of curricular reform.

These reforms went hand in hand with those occurring in American collegiate education. Post–World War II America was committed to broadening access to higher education for all its citizens. President Harry Truman's Commission on Higher Education pointed to a substantially broadened network of community colleges awarding associate degrees as the critical component of this agenda. Each such college would be deeply situated within and oriented toward the needs of its community. It would attract its students from its community, provide them with easy access to a modestly priced education, and return them to their communities armed with the knowledge and the technical expertise to meet local needs. Community colleges would also provide a new form of higher education to men and women without the material or social resources necessary to attend a traditional four-year college or university. On the one hand, this would broaden the educational opportunities available to working-class men and women. On the other hand, it would relieve the pressures placed by these same men and women, many of them veterans armed with educational funding from the GI Bill, for access to a limited number of more prestigious places in traditional colleges and universities. For some community college graduates, their vocationally oriented associate degree would provide a springboard to a place within colleges emphasizing the liberal arts and sciences. For many more others, it would provide a valued credential that testified to certain concrete skills and knowledge.

American nursing leaders, hoping to break the stranglehold of service-oriented hospital-based programs on nursing education, eyed such opportunities in community colleges with interest. Their idea was that these programs would create a hierarchical system of practice and authority within nursing. With the implicit acknowledgment that an associate degree stood as a code word for a working-class individual's opportunity, such a two-year graduate would be recognized as a "technical nurse," always working under the direction of a "professional nurse" with a more substantive educational background. But graduates of community college nursing programs sat for the same registration exam as did those of the most prestigious collegiate nursing programs. And under the press of day-to-day hospital practice, they soon proved themselves as competent.

The numbers of these associate degree programs rose exponentially from seven in the early 1950s to almost seven hundred in the mid-1970s. Community college presidents welcomed the prestige that accompanied their establishment. The women and, increasingly, the men in their local communities welcomed the opportunities.[28] There were now three ways to become a registered nurse: through traditional, although rapidly disappearing hospital-based diploma programs; through collegiate programs that were increasingly located in freestanding schools within universities, rather than the earlier amalgam of hospital training followed by university coursework; and through more accessible community colleges.

Nurses: More and More Diversity

Changes in practice patterns, funding opportunities, and curricular structures affected the numbers of American nurses. The numbers leaped 118 percent in the 1950s, before settling to fairly stable advances of 25 to 35 percent each decade through the close of the twentieth century. But more dramatic changes occurred within nursing. Even as the absolute numbers of white female nurses grew, nursing was less and less exclusively white and less and less exclusively women's work. In 1950, 98 percent of all nurses were women, and 94 percent were white women. By 1970, nursing was still predominantly women's work, but only 90 percent of female nurses were white. The numbers continued to plummet. By 1990, women represented 95 percent of all nurses, and only 81 percent of all nurses were white women. By 2006, only 92 percent of all nurses were women, and only 74 percent of nurses were white women. In terms of blunt demographics, nursing had returned to those surrounding its late nineteenth-century birth, where, in 1900, women represented 91 percent of all nurses, and white women represented 89 percent of such women (Table A.2).

The numbers of white and African American men who identified as nurses grew during this period. But the most dramatic proportionate increases came from women and men with non-white and non–African American backgrounds (Table A.1). The absolute numbers remained relatively small compared to white and African American nurses; and the census sampling precludes reliably identifying these nurses as other than non-white and non–African American. However, national sample surveys of registered nurses found that these women were predominately of Asian, Pacific Islander, and Hispanic descent.

Many of these non-white and non–African American nurses had been born and educated in the Philippines. As Catherine Cenzia Choy points out in her history of Filipino nurse migration to the United States, the relationships among these women and American nurses had deep and tangled roots. Even as white American nursing leaders excluded most African American women from their schools in the early twentieth century, and even as they worried about the slipping place of white middle-class women in the images of nursing's work, they were traveling to the Philippines, then an American colony, to establish training schools and to encourage young Filipino women to become nurses. Certainly, as Choy argues, this seeming benevolence has to be understood in the context of American imperialism. But in the face of the critical nursing shortages of the postwar era, the Americanized training models—as well as cold war politics, changes in immigration policies, and the Philippine government's institutionalization of nursing and nurses as a critical component of its export economy—set the stage for the waves of Filipino nurse immigration in the latter half of the twentieth century.[29]

Filipino women and others from different non-white and non–African American backgrounds were slowly changing the face of nursing. Those identifying as professional nurses represented less than 1 percent of all nurses in 1950. Yet by 2006, they represented 9 percent of all nurses and 10 percent of all female nurses. We know much less about non-white and non–African American men. The census data show that those identifying as professional nurses came into nursing later. Their numbers grew more substantially after 1970 (Table A.1). By 2006, men had regained their 1900 place in nursing. Male nurses of color had a stronger presence vis-à-vis male nurses than did women of color. Twenty-six percent of male nurses were those of color (Table A.2).

Some small numbers of American-born, non-white and non–African American women, well-known in their local communities although almost completely invisible to their broader nursing community, had always practiced as registered nurses. Like some white and African American colleagues, some were also discouraged from becoming nurses. For example, Louise Smith, later acknowledged by white colleagues as the first trained Hopi Indian nurse, remembered that her tribe disapproved of her ambitions to train as a nurse in the 1920s because of its concern over her "catching" the white man's illnesses and about learning the "white man's ways." Like many of her American nursing colleagues who also felt little family or community support, Smith's ideas about working as a nurse developed during direct contact with one who had cared for her during recurring episodes of a chronic eye infection. "I never took my eyes off her," Smith recalled, "and she was my model."

But like Ludie Andrews and Annie Feebeck at Grady Hospital in Atlanta, Smith always remained aware that her ambition for herself lay within a racialized context. She might learn to cook from the wife of the local Bureau of Indian Affairs superintendent or learn to nurse with white students at the Methodist Hospital School of Nursing in Los Angeles, where she graduated in 1927. But racial barriers remained as high for nurses like Smith as it did for their African American colleagues. Smith had to fight the white nursing administration to receive the same civil service status and security that her white colleagues enjoyed at the Tuba City Hospital where she worked. It was a difficult battle with little community support. Smith won such status only after successfully recruiting outside allies from Washington, D.C.'s Bureau of Indian Affairs, the federal department that ran the hospital.[30]

Other such nurses were relatively well known and well respected within their particular communities, and they had their communities' support in their battles to become nurses. Minnie Fong Lee, recognized as the first Chinese American woman to become a public health nurse in California in 1931, found herself inspired to consider nursing "by a very lovely school nurse, a sort of heroine to me." Stanford University School of Nursing refused to consider her application because she was Asian, but the school at the San Francisco General Hospital did admit her. Her dream was to become a public health nurse, and she worked hard, taking the necessary courses at the University of California at Berkeley by day, and working at the Chinese Hospital in San Francisco by night. Lee, however, found herself barred from taking the exam because, at barely over five feet in height, she failed to meet the minimum height requirement of five feet and two inches—a standard that had long served as a white barrier to Chinese women who wished to work as public health nurses. But Lee came from a strongly supportive family and community. Her sister, Alice Fong Yu, had already battled for and won a position as the first Chinese public school teacher in San Francisco. Her community's Chinese Six Companies and the Chinese American Citizen's Alliance also had a strong commitment to the political rights and the social ambitions of its members. "They all went to bat for me," Lee remembered, and the height requirement was removed from the list of qualifications.[31]

Crossing the Class Divide

Like their early twentieth-century counterparts at St. Luke's and Lincoln Hospitals in New York City and at the Latter Day Saints Hospital in Salt Lake City, some later twentieth-century nurses did come from the kinds of middle-class social and secure backgrounds envisioned by American nursing leaders as representative of an ideal nurse. But many more came from different social, racial, and economic backgrounds. Like other nurses, these women and men came to nursing with intellect, ambition, and aspirations for themselves and sometimes for the social groups they represented. They may have mythologized the white Florence Nightingale, but they also appropriated that same myth's power in the construction of meaningful and deeply held identities as nurses. Nursing provided few guarantees—few promises that their sense of themselves would be consistently recognized by others and few assurances that their work would have its own material rewards. But it did provide concrete markers of content and character that could be a pass-port across the class divide in their particular communities.

This use of work as a means across the class divide was not, of course, unique to nursing. In ways constantly repeated in the history of women and work, where middle-class women went first, working-class women soon followed. Domestic service, for example, was initially the domain of young, "middling" girls, apprenticed to learn the necessary house-keeping skills; immigrant and African American women soon followed. Women of "good Yankee stock" first worked the looms of nineteenth-century American textile mills; poor, working-class women also soon followed. But when immigrant and African American women entered domestic service, "middling" girls fled. When poor and working class women entered the mills, Yankee women abandoned them.[32] Yet white, middle-class flight, to the profession's credit, did not occur in nursing. It did not occur at St. Luke's in New York City when the demand for nurses had surged in the early twentieth century. And it did not occur later, as African American, American Indian, Chinese American, Hispanic and Latino Americans, and Asian Americans became more and more visible as they trained and practiced as nurses throughout the later twentieth century. As in North Carolina, a strong professional identity; real op-portunities for talented and ambitious persons of all classes, races, and gender; as well as stratified patterns of education and practice have kept all groups tied together tightly—albeit, as in Georgia, not always easily—throughout its history.

But the meaning of the work did play out differently for different nurses. While patterns of work and marital status may have been virtu-ally indistinguishable among white and African American female nurses in 1940, differences began appearing in 1960 that gained momentum through the succeeding decades. African American female nurses living with their spouses began leaving the nursing workforce at rates much higher than those of white women, nurses from other racial backgrounds, and white men. And while marital status among white women, women from non-white and non–African American backgrounds, and white men converged in the 1980s (Table A.4a), those of married African American women living with their husbands plummeted to 48 percent in 1980, to 45 percent in 2000, and to 41 percent in 2006 (Figure 7.3). We see, in fact, a complete reversal of early twentieth-century trends in

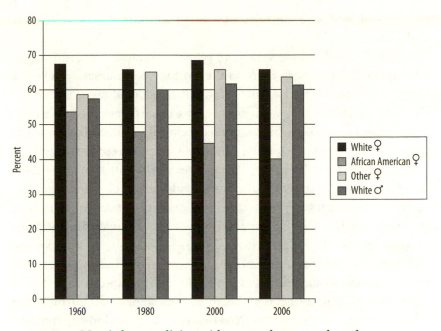

FIGURE 7.3. Married nurses living with spouses by race and gender.
Source: Table A.4a.

identification as nurses and marital status for African American women. Whereas married African American nurses living with their spouses once had higher workforce participation rates than white female nurses, they now have significantly lower ones.

The ages of married female and male nurses living with their spouses (rather than separated from them) is significant as an explanation. In 1980, only 24 percent of married African American female nurses living with their spouses were under forty years of age, as compared to 39 percent of comparable white women, 46 percent of other women of color, and 41 percent of white men (Table A.5). This trend continued through 2000 and, in fact, heightened as the African American women identifying as nurses aged. By 2000, only 33 percent of married African American female nurses living with spouses and under the age of fifty remained in the workforce, as compared to 49 percent of comparable white women and other nurses of color, and 48 percent white men (Table A.5). These age ranges, of course, correspond with those within which women and men were most likely to start their families and raise their children.

Other national sample surveys of registered nurses have repeatedly documented the withdrawal from the workforce of nurses with young children at home. They have not, however, considered racial dynamics. Census data, by contrast, highlight the importance of race. African American female nurses did remain more economically vulnerable than white nurses, other nurses of color, and white men in instances when, by choice or by circumstance, they found themselves as the sole support of their own families as separated from spouses, widowed, or divorced. As in the early twentieth century, these women show higher rates of workforce participation than their colleagues. The situation changed dramatically, however, when they found themselves in partnership with spouses. These married African American women may have chosen to move out of nursing and assume different kinds of identities and to do different kinds of work. But the fact that this trend persisted, that it mirrored the well-documented aging of the American nursing workforce, and that data show some of these women returning to nursing when their marital circumstances changed strongly suggest another possibility. These African American women's intellect, ambitions, and aspirations had their own meaningful and tangible reward. Those particularly positioned and who so chose could attain the historically elusive goal of raising their own rather than other women's children.

Crossing the Educational Divide

Family and family life remained important. But these were only some components of lives as nurses. Education was equally important. Through the 1960s, a nursing credential assured its holder of a place among the more educated of all American women. All nurses, for example, needed at least a high school education for entry into diploma, associate degree, or bachelor's degree programs, but only 55 percent of all American women could claim such a credential.[33] Still, a college or university experience was often an ambitious and sometimes elusive goal for both female and male nurses. A sizeable number of female nurses did succeed in gaining a bachelor's degree in nursing as their first professional credential. The numbers increased from 13 percent in 1960 to 31 percent in

2004. But at the same time, the numbers of American women earning bachelor's degrees as their initial collegiate degree soared from 8 percent in 1960 to 32 percent in 2004. By this measure, American nurses found themselves, for the first time, at a distinct disadvantage, given the place of education as a proxy for class and community standing (Figure 7.4).

Some American nursing leaders re-sounded the alarm. In 1998, Luther Christman, the first male dean of nursing, first at Vanderbilt University School of Nursing and later at Rush University's College of Nursing, wrote a scorching critique of what he saw as the failure of American nursing to seize the opportunity to definitively establish the bachelor's degree as the only pathway to professional nursing practice. Appalling disciplinary apathy and troubling gender homogeneity, he argued, only perpetuated and never resolved the unending dilemma of three entry levels into the profession. And three entry levels at the diploma, associate degree, and bachelor's level, he continued, ruined

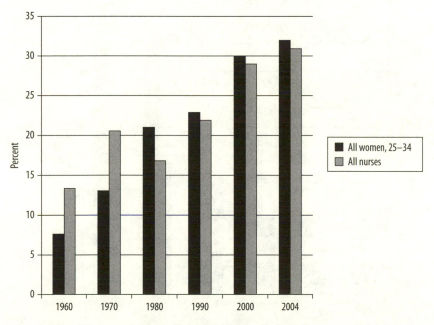

FIGURE 7.4. Women 25–34 and nurses with bachelor's degrees as initial professional credential. *Source:* Table A.6.

nursing's image in the media. Why, Christman queried, should we expect our image to be otherwise? *"Nurses insist,"* he stated in italics for emphasis, *"on being the poorest prepared of all the professions."*[34]

Yet Christman's picture of preparedness dramatically changes when one turns from considering the numbers of nurses earning bachelor's degrees as their first professional credential to those who eventually earn such a degree over a lifetime of practice. The numbers of nurses earning a bachelor's degree or higher over a lifetime rose from 9 percent in 1960 to 47 percent in 2004. American nurses may have entered their working lives at an educational disadvantage when compared to American women in general. But they have refused to stay there. The proportion of American nurses who have earned a bachelor's degree over their lifetime far exceeds that of American women in general through 2004 (Figure 7.5).

The advantages accrued to American nurses of color are even more pronounced. Because the numbers of non-white women who achieved

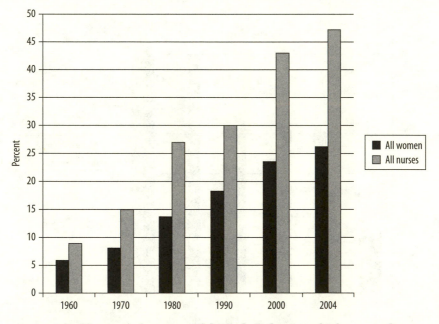

FIGURE 7.5. Women and nurses with bachelor's degree or higher earned over a lifetime. *Source:* Table A.7.

bachelor degrees in any field over their lifetime remained relatively low prior to the civil rights movement of the 1960s and 1970s, such early data need to be treated cautiously. But national sample survey data from both 2000 and 2004 suggest that the current proportion of nurses of color with bachelor's degrees earned over a lifetime is greater than that of white nurses. The absolute numbers remain smaller than those of white nurses, still the predominant group of American nurses. But in 2004, only 46 percent of white nurses had earned a bachelor's degree at some point in their lives. By contrast, 52 percent of African American nurses and 72 percent of Asian or Pacific Islander nurses could point to such an accomplishment. Hispanic nurses match their white colleagues at 46 percent (Figure 7.6).

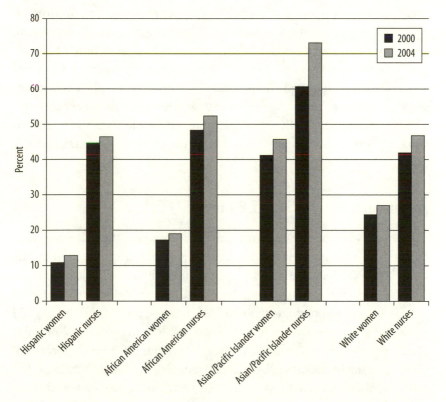

FIGURE 7.6. Women and nurses with bachelor's degree or higher earned over a lifetime, by race. *Source:* Table A.8.

Most nurses of color were also substantially more educated than other women in their own racial or ethnic communities than white nurses were in their communities. Again in 2004, 52 percent of African American nurses earned a bachelor's degree at some point in their life, compared to 19 percent of all African American women. Similarly, 46 percent of Hispanic nurses earned bachelor's degrees, yet only 12 percent of other such women did. The numbers are less dramatic but still substantive for Asian and Pacific Islander nurses, despite the fact that many received their initial nursing education in the Philippines, where the bachelor's degree was the only pathway to practice. Seventy-three percent of Asian and Pacific Islander nurses held a bachelor's degree; 46 percent of women in the Asian and Pacific Islander community did (Figure 7.6).

Still, as Jerome Lysaught first pointed out in 1973, the social and economic successes in terms of bachelor's degrees earned over a lifetime for all nurses has come at an enormously high personal, emotional, social, and financial cost to nurses.[35] These women and men built their degrees course by course, year in and year out, as they continued to work as nurses. Some received small subsidies from their employers to cover some of the costs. But in the end, nurses and their families were the ones who bore the burden of their considerable achievements as the historical trade of work for knowledge played itself out in its twenty-first-century form.

Rethinking the Work and Worth of Nursing

The actual work of nursing—the skilled body work, the intimate emotional demands, and the managing of the boundaries between public and private worlds—remains as trying and often as difficult today as it was in the nineteenth century. In 2004, for example, those national sample survey respondents who had left nursing reported that they did so because of stressful work environments, long hours, and low salaries.[36] Still, 76 percent of those nurses who remained, and 74 percent of those working in the most direct and intense hospital staff nursing roles, also described themselves as moderately or extremely satisfied with their positions.[37] One might consider those who left for other possibilities as replicating longstanding historical patterns of resourcefulness and adaptability. Those who remain to do the work of nursing still see themselves as doing valuable and valued work.

Yet these ideas would be framed by a traditional perspective that considers nursing only in relation to their actual work. Nursing, as we have seen, is not just about the work: it is also about the meaning of the work. These meanings have often been about class and community status. They have been about who had a place within and who aspired to a particular social group. Unlike most other accessible kinds of work, nursing provided opportunities to many from a variety of backgrounds seeking a step up from and out of traditional expectations. Many different individuals at different times with different places in their own communities of family, friends, and colleagues chose to do the work of nursing with very different dreams and aspirations.

Certainly, most women and men who chose to do nursing's work wanted to do good. But they also wanted to do well. And they have wanted to do so in the social spaces they occupied in their own communities, neighborhoods, professional organizations, and families as well as in the clinical spaces that these many different men and women created in their workplaces. The women and some men who chose to do the work of nursing understood the enduring link between education and at least the perception of middle-class community status in twentieth-century America. Whether they chose nursing as a lifelong commitment to a kind of work or as a strategic plan that moved them toward the creation of a different kind of life, they always believed that an identity as a nurse gave them, both by association and by virtue of their special training, a place among the more-educated members of particular—albeit not all—communities.

One might delve more deeply into such meanings by considering one striking change between the nineteenth and twenty-first centuries. Nurses are now no longer the only women with legitimate claims to medical knowledge. The numbers of women seeking careers as physicians have grown steadily since the 1960s. Women now number almost 28 percent of the physician workforce, and medical school classes now approach 50 percent women students.[38] Yet as one claim slipped away, another surfaced. Nurses may no longer be the only women (and they themselves may not only be women) with such claims, but they are the ones whose claims to such are most trusted by the American public. Since 1999, when nursing was first added to the Gallup's annual survey of professions, the men and women who do its work have consistently been voted the country's most honest and ethical professionals. There was one exception. In 2001, firefighters took pride of place in the aftermath of 9/11. The leadership of the American Nurses Association has always characterized this achievement as emblematic of nurses' relationships with the individual patients they treat. But nursing's resurgence and persistence also reflects its articulation of a more fundamental relationship among knowledge, identity, and social place that remains fairly constant over time. Nurses have always been in and of their particularly diverse communities, leaving for work opportunities, sometimes returning to them in marriage and parenthood, and often serving within them as models of opportunity for other women and men. The specialized skill, the disciplined persona, the deep commitment, and the relatively privileged position that nurses hold have always and still do carry powerful meanings.

Historically, these meanings were most often gendered. They celebrated the women that these nurses were. But they also celebrated the women that they wanted to become. A formal nursing identity—that is, a gendered identity built around the social salience of a particular kind of work—enabled women and some men to create a more coherent and a more sustained independent place for themselves within their chosen sphere. It gave individuals the power to renegotiate the terms of some of the inequities they experienced and to shape their own sense of the value of work in their lives. It may not always have done so in ways that met their expectations. But it did create a broader range of opportunities at particular points in time and over the course of a lifetime.

Some of these opportunities were quite personal. Nursing allowed women working within different religious and racial traditions to construct lives that reflected their own personal commitments to individual self-fulfillment and to the needs of their families. Others were quite political. Nursing allowed other women to make powerful statements about race and class that flew in the face of social perceptions. It created traditions of access and opportunity now open to men as well as women. Certainly, as this history of nurses and nursing has suggested, there are significant problems when this deeply internalized identity finds little validation in the wider world. But when one shifts the perspective from work to the meaning of the work to lives lived in families, communities, and, for some, on a broader national stage, one also sees substantive possibilities inherent in the work and worth of nursing.

D ATA COME from the Integrated Public Use Microdata Series (IPUMS-USA).[1] IPUMS data draw on thirty-nine high-precision samples of the American population drawn from fifteen federal censuses and from the American Community Surveys of 2000–2006 (http://usa.ipums.org/usa/index .shtml). Sample size is 1 percent from 1900 to 1970 and 5 percent from 1980 to 2000. IPUMS samples the American Community Survey for 2006 data.

The estimation of registered (or professional) nurse was selected from the IPUMS variable P OCC1950 058 professional-nurses. OCC1950 applies the 1950 Census Bureau's occupational classification system to all occupational data to enhance comparability across the years. The design of OCC1950 is described at length at http://usa.ipums.org/usa-action/variableDescription.do?mnemonic= OCC1950. Since the IPUM's occupational variable captures self-identification, it does overstate the absolute numbers of registered professional nurses.

The category "professional nurse" can be a constantly shifting one. Therefore, demographic data from 1970 through the present were also collected using the IPUMS OCC1990 095 category "registered nurse." Like OCC1950, OCC1990 offers researchers a consistent long-term classification of occupations, but for methodological reasons it is preferred for samples from 1970 onward. In this analysis, the OCC1990 categorization brought the overall estimates of registered nurses more in line with other data sources, including the national sample surveys of registered nurses. However, the OCC1990 within group proportional estimates remained virtually identical to those of the OCC1950. Data for 1960 remained identical for both OCC1950 and OCC1990 estimates, making it a good bridge between the different bases of analyses.

The categorization of race is particularly problematic since the concept and the categories have constantly changed over the more than 150 years

---

[1]Steven Ruggles, Matthew Sobek, Trent Alexander, Catherine A. Fitch, Ronald Goeken, Patricia Kelly Hall, Miriam King, and Chad Ronnander, *Integrated Public Use Microdata Series: Version 4.0* (machine-readable database) (Minneapolis: Minnesota Population Center [producer and distributor], 2008).

represented in the IPUMS sample. The IPUMS 1 percent and 5 percent samples yield too few estimates of the particular groups of non-white, non–African American women and men who identified as nurses in the latter half of the twentieth century for reliable inferences. This analysis, by necessity, groups them together when considering patterns of change over time and limits its analyses to those that have the most sampled data: white women, African American women, other women of color, and white men. Also, the groupings of racial and ethnic categories have changed and only recently acknowledge multiracial backgrounds. Given such issues, this analysis uses IPUMS race categories as only a broad measure of the percentages of non-white and non–African American nurses. More specific analyses of race draw from the periodic national surveys done of the registered nurse population in the later twentieth century.

Finally, the IPUMS assumes a correlation between occupational identification and workforce participation. The 1950 occupational standardization uses census criteria that ask for occupational data only if one is presently in the workforce. But caution is also needed because there is no differentiation made between those who may have had a full-time position and those with part-time or intermittent periods of employment. This analysis, though, is less interested in actual numbers of nurses and more interested in how the proportions of nurse within one gender or race category compares with those of others at particular points in time. It is as interested in significant trends over time. For all its limitations, the IPUMS data remain, to date, the only source of information about the trends of gender, race, and social place. The IPUMS data does trend in ways that are consistent with other studies about white nurses' workforce participation. May Ayres Burgess's 1928 survey, for example, shows life-cycle patterns similar to that of IPUMS.[2] And later twentieth-century census data also trend in ways that are consistent with national sample survey data that document the increasing opportunities nursing offered to white women, to nurses of color, and to men.

[2] May Ayres Burgess, *Nurses, Patients, and Pocketbooks: A Study of the Economics of Nursing by the Committee on the Grading of Nursing Schools* (New York: Committee on the Grading of Nursing Schools, 1928), 49–55.

TABLE A.1 Professional nurses, by gender and race, 1900–2006 (as total self-identifying)

Year	Total nurses	% increase	Total men	White men	African American men	Other men	Total women	White women	African American women	Other women
1900	10,833		1,000	800	200		9,833	9,632	201	
1910	73,917	582	4,210	4,009	201		69,707	66,596	3,010	101
1920	116,965	58	4,440	4,339	101		112,525	109,296	2,927	302
1930	230,482	97	5,656	5,353	101	202	224,826	218,766	5,454	606
1940	340,025	47	12,561	12,461	100		327,464	319,303	7,361	800
1950	415,439	22	9,489	8,818	671		405,950	391,435	13,236	1,279
1960	905,914	118	15,340	13,150	1,893	297	890,574	841,784	42,419	6,371
1970[a]	1,218,400	35	29,900	25,300	3,800	800	1,188,500	1,096,200	69,400	22,900
1980[a]	1,547,360	27	58,500	49,500	6,360	2,640	1,488,860	1,330,360	102,680	55,820
1990[a]	2,151,486	39	113,401	93,656	11,334	8,411	2,038,085	1,749,979	176,311	111,795
2000[a]	2,648,666	23	189,459	148,385	16,636	24,438	2,459,207	2,026,210	222,169	210,828
2006[a]	2,889,576		248,237	184,154	24,943	39,040	2,641,339	2,127,957	252,211	261,119

SOURCE: Integrated Public Use Microdata Series (IPUMS-USA) available at http://usa.ipums.org/usa/index.shtml.
[a]These percents calculated using the OCC1990 as a more reliable estimate of numbers of nurses.

TABLE A.2 Professional nurses, by gender and race, 1900–2006 (as percentages)

Year	Total men	White men as % of all nurses	White men as % of all men	African American men as % of all men	Other men as % of all men	Total women	White women as % of all nurses	White women as % of all women	African American women as % of all women	Other women as % of all women
1900	9	7	80	10		91	89	98	2	
1910	6	5	95	5		94	90	95	4	1
1920	3.7	4	98	2		96	93	97	2.6	<1
1930	2.4	2	95	2	3	98	95	97	2.4	<1
1940	4	3.6	99	<1		96	94	96	3	<1
1950	2	2	93	7		98	94	96	3	<1
1960	2	1.5	86	12	2	98	93	94	5	<1
1970[a]	2.5	2.1	85	13	3	97.5	90	92	6	5
1980[a]	4	3.2	85	11	5	96	86	89	7	4
1990[a]	5.3	4.4	83	10	6	95	81	86	8.5	5.5
2000[a]	7.2	5.6	78	9	13	93	76	82	9	9
2006[a]	8.6	6.4	74	10	16	92	74	80	10	10

SOURCE: Integrated Public Use Microdata Series (IPUMS-USA) available at http://usa.ipums.org/usa/index.shtml.

[a]These percentages calculated using the OCC1990 as a more reliable estimate of numbers of nurses. Total slightly exceeds 100 percent because of rounding issues.

TABLE A.3   Men practical nurses, by race

Year	Total men	White men	African American men	African American men as % of all men
1900	6,514	5,612	902	14
1910	3,909	3,009	900	23
1920	4,139	3,531	608	2
1930	3,030	2,727	303	1
1940	7,232	6,274	958	13
1950	5,747	5,087	660	12
1960	12,148	10,353	1,794	15
1970	11,400	8,300	3,100	27
1980	16,520	13,320	3,200	20
1990	27,928	21,178	6,749	24
2000	41,591	30,336	11,255	27
2006	51,729	36,981	14,748	29

SOURCE: Integrated Public Use Microdata Series (IPUMS-USA) available at http://usa.ipums.org/usa/index.shtml.

TABLE A.4 Nurses' marital status, by race and gender (as total self-identifying)

	Single				Married—spouse present			
Year	White women	African American women	Other women	White men	White women	African American women	Other women	White men
1900	9,126				301	201		
1920	91,230	1,513			5,249	606		
1930	158,772	2,323			26,664	1,414		
1940	219,178	4,606		3,853	56,545	1,515		7,108
1950	156,055	4,196		2,129	163,829	5,138		4,577
1960	150,516	7,769	1,489	3,087	572,931	23,100	4,085	7,575
1970[b]	174,300	9,800		8,300	743,500	38,000		13,000
1980[b]	230,840	20,360	13,020	14,220	880,940	49,780	35,120	29,320
1990[b]	227,582	38,544		22,963	1,198,584	75,370		58,762
2000[b]	210,307	47,223	32,948	33,190	1,406,459	100,597	140,384	92,268
2006[b]	251,292	66,599	43,390	38,894	10,404,141	104,054	168,063	113,476

SOURCE: Integrated Public Use Microdata Series (IPUMS-USA) available at http://usa.ipums.org/usa/index.shtml.

[a]Includes those who indicated they had separated from their spouses.

[b]Calculated using the OCC1990 as a more reliable estimate of numbers of nurses.

TABLE A.4A Nurses' marital status, by race and gender (as percentages)

	Single				Married—spouse present			
Year	White women	African American women	Other women	White men	White women	African American women	Other women	White men
1920	83	52			5	21		
1930	73	43			12	26		
1940	68	63		31	18	21		57
1950	40	32		24	42	39		52
1960	18	18	23	24	68	54	59	58
1970[b]	16	14		33	68	55		26
1980[b]	17	20	23	29	66	48	65	60
1990[b]	13	22		24	68	43		63
2000[b]	10	21	16	22	69	45	66	62
2006[b]	12	26	18	21	66	41	64	62

SOURCE: Integrated Public Use Microdata Series (IPUMS-USA) available at http://usa.ipums.org/usa/index.shtml.

[a]Includes those who indicated they had separated from their spouses.

[b]These percentages were calculated using the OCC1990 as a more reliable estimate of numbers of nurses.

Married—spouse absent[a]				Widowed				Divorced			
White women	African American women	Other women	White men	White women	African American women	Other women	White men	White women	African American women	Other women	White men
402				603							
3,834	404			6,862	404			2,121			
8,787	505			19,291	1,212			5,252			
12,535	600		700	20,075	200		700	10,270	400		100
20,811	2,165		1,221	28,823	1,506		396	21,917	231		495
23,803	5,476	698	1,093	62,257	3,485	99	896	32,277	2,589	0	599
32,900	8,000		1,000	92,500	7,200		1,000	53,000	6,400		2,000
29,560	10,200	2,860	1,680	72,340	5,900	1,320	340	115,680	16,440	2,480	3,940
41,158	18,563		2,884	76,770	11,160		621	205,885	32,674		8,246
50,269	20,193	12,120	4,379	73,179	13,320	4,923	865	285,966	40,936	20,453	17,685
63,206	22,702	18,759	5,840	76,295	10,876	7,424	2,614	333,003	47,992	23,556	23,430

Married—spouse absent[a]				Widowed				Divorced			
White women	African American women	Other women	White men	White women	African American women	Other women	White men	White women	African American women	Other women	White men
4	14			6	14			2	0		
4	10			9	22			2	0		
4	8		6	7	5		6	3	3		<1
5.3	16		14	7	11		4	4	2		6
3	13	11	8	8	8	1	7		6	0	4
3	12		3	8.4	10		3	5	9		8
2.3	10	5	3	5.5	5.8	2	1	9	16	4	8
2	10		3	4	6		1	12	18		8
2.5	9	6	3	4	5.2	2.4	1	14	18	10	11
3	9	7	3	4	4	3	1	12	19	9	13

TABLE A.5 Nurses living with spouses, by age, race, and gender, 1980 and 2000 (as total self-identifying and as percentages)

	1980								2000							
	White women		African American women		Other women		White men		White women		African American women		Other women		White men	
Age	N	%	N	%	N	%	N	%	N	%	N	%	N	%	N	%
5–19	360	<1	100	<1	20	<1	20	<1	153	<1	25	<1	18	<1		<1
20–24	66,700	5	2,200	2	700	1	1,620	3	21,464	1	1,324	1	1,449	1	1,212	1
25–29	172,800	13	7,900	8	5,600	10	7,560	15	107,067	5	6,256	3	11,426	5	7,945	5
30–34	152,520	11	8,720	8	10,400	19	7,680	16	151,427	7	12,626	6	19,965	9	12,931	9
35–39	115,680	9	8,080	8	8,720	16	3,620	7	223,398	11	18,552	8	20,737	10	16,126	11
40–44	95,780	7	7,200	7	4,820	9	2,126	4	264,641	13	18,746	8	27,604	13	17,079	12
45–49	87,080	7	6,200	6	3,120	6	1,800	4	239,534	12	15,517	7	24,849	12	17,622	12
50–54	74,320	6	4,380	4	1,200	2	1,600	3	168,149	8	11,433	5	16,376	8	11,198	8
55–59	61,080	5	2,760	3	1,020	2	1,100	2	114,479	6	7,833	4	10,224	5	4,641	3
60–64	34,500	3	1,300	1	240	<1	1,120	2	67,638	3	4,672	2	5,257	2	2,296	2
>65	21,120	2	940	1	300	<1	920	2	48,509	2	3,615	2	2,479	1	1,218	1
Total	880,940		49,780		35,120		29,320		1,406,459		100,597		140,384		92,268	

SOURCE: Integrated Public Use Microdata Series (IPUMS-USA) available at http://usa.ipums.org/usa/index.shtml.
For 1980: N all white women nurses = 1,330,360; N all African American women nurses = 102,680; N all other women nurses = 55,820; N all white men nurses = 49,500.
For 2000: N all white women nurses = 2,026,210; N all African American women nurses = 222,169; N all other women nurses = 210,828; N all white men nurses = 148,385.

TABLE A.6   U.S. women aged 25–34 and nurses with bachelor's degrees as initial professional credential (as percentages)

	1960	1970	1980	1990	2000	2004
All women, 25–34	7.5	13	21	23	30	32
All nurses	13.4	20.8	17	22	29	31

SOURCE: U.S. Census Table A-1, "Years of School Completed by People 25 Years and Over, by Age and Sex: Selected Years 1940-2007 (www.census.gov/population/www/socdemo/educ-attn.html).

NOTE: This table concentrates on data in Table A-1 on women between 25 and 34 as that most comparable to nurses who tended to be between 24 and 28 when they received their initial bachelor's degree (see *National Sample Survey 2002*, p. 25). *The Sourcebook: Nursing Personnel (1974)*, p. 69 showed data on nurses 1952–1974; *The National Sample Survey of Registered Nurses 2002* (http://bhpr.hrsa.gov/healthworkforce/reports/rnsurvey/rnss1.htm) showed data on nurses 1980–2000; and the *National Sample Survey of Registered Nurses 2004* (http://bhpr.hrsa.gov/healthworkforce/rnsurvey04/preface.htm) provided that for 2004.

TABLE A.7   U.S. women and nurses with bachelor's degrees or higher earned over a lifetime (as percentages)

	1960	1970	1980	1990	2000	2004
All women	5.8	8.2	13.6	18.4	23.6	26.1
All nurses	9.1	14.8	27	30	42.9	47.2

SOURCE: U.S. Census Table A-1; *The Sourcebook: Nursing Personnel (1974)*, p. 69, showed data on nurses 1952–1974; *The National Sample Survey 2002* showed data on nurses 1980–2000; and the *National Sample Survey 2004* provided that for 2004.

TABLE A.8   U.S. women and nurses with bachelor's degrees or higher earned over a lifetime, by race (as percentages)

	2000	*2004*
Hispanic women	10.6	12.3
Hispanic nurses	44.6	46.4
African American women	16.7	18.5
African American nurses	48.1	52
Asian/Pacific Islander women	40.7	45.6
Asian/Pacific Islander nurses	60.5	72.6
White women	23.9	26.4
White nurses	41.8	46.5

SOURCE: For data on women by race, see census data No. 222 Educational Attainment by Race, Hispanic Origin, and Sex 1960 to 2007 (www.census.gov/compendia/statab/tables/ 09s0222.pdf). *The National Sample Survey 2002* showed data on nurses in 2000, and the *National Sample Survey 2004* provided that for 2004.

Chapter One: Nurses and Physicians in Nineteenth-Century Philadelphia

1. For Phillips's Woman's Hospital career, see Minutes of the Board of Managers, Woman's Hospital of Philadelphia, January 1872 and September 1872, Archives and Special Collections of Women in Medicine and Homeopathy, Drexel University College of Medicine. For her work at the Chinese Mission Home, see Peggy Pascoe, *Relations of Rescue: The Search for Female Moral Authority in the American West, 1874–1939* (New York: Oxford University Press, 1990), 77.

2. Bancroft Library, University of California, Berkeley, Children's Hospital of San Francisco Papers 1875–1978, MSS 89/87C, carton 10, folder 10.7

3. Gail Farr Casterline, "Ellis R. Shipp," in *Sister Saints*, ed. Vicky Burgess-Olson (Ogden, UT: Brigham Young University Press, 1975), 365–81.

4. Minutes of the Board of Managers, Woman's Hospital of Philadelphia, January 1872 and September 1872, Archives and Special Collections of Women in Medicine and Homeopathy, Drexel University College of Medicine. For a consideration of the role of the Woman's Hospital in the development of nursing in the United States, see Patricia O'Brien, "'All a Woman's Life Can Bring': The Domestic Roots of Nursing in Philadelphia, 1830–1885," *Nursing Research* 36, no. 1 (1987): 12–17.

5. For a review, see Philip A. Kalisch and Beatrice J. Kalisch, *The Advance of American Nursing*, 3rd ed. (Philadelphia: J. B. Lippincott, 1995), 57–73.

6. See analysis in Miriam Bailin, *The Sickroom in Victorian Fiction: The Art of Being Ill* (New York: Cambridge University Press, 1994). See also Judith Flanders, *The Victorian House: Domestic Life from Childbirth to Deathbed* (New York: HarperCollins, 2003), 302–48.

7. Emily Abel, *Hearts of Wisdom: American Women Caring for Kin, 1850–1940* (Cambridge, MA: Harvard University Press, 2000).

8. *Sick Chamber*, (no author) (Boston: James Munroe and Co., 1847), 5.

9. Ibid., 17–31.

10. See, for example, Linda Sabin, "Unheralded Nurses: Male Caregivers in the 19th Century South," *Nursing History Review* 5 (1997): 131–48.

11. Patricia D'Antonio, "The Legacy of Domesticity: Nursing in Early 19th Century America," *Nursing History Review* 1 (1993): 229–46. See also Lamar Riley Murphy, *Enter the Physician: The Transformation of Domestic Medicine, 1760–1860* (Tuscaloosa: University of Alabama Press, 1991)

12. Kathleen Brown, "The Maternal Physician: Teaching Mothers to Put the Baby in the Bathwater," in *Right Living: An Anglo-American Tradition of Self-Help Medicine and Hygiene,* ed. Charles Rosenberg (Baltimore: Johns Hopkins University Press, 2003), 88–111; James C. Whorton, *Nature Cures: The History of Alternative Medicine in America* (New York: Oxford University Press, 2002).

13. Anthony Todd Thomson, *The Domestic Management of the Sick Room, Necessary in Aid of Medical Treatment, for the Cure of Diseases* (Philadelphia: Lea & Blanchard, 1845), 105.

14. Lydia Child, *The Family Nurse or Companion of the American Frugal Housewife* (Boston: Charles J. Hinde, 1837).

15. "Florence Nightingale's Book," *Godey's Lady's Book and Magazine* 61 (September 1860): 269.

16. Review in *The Quarterly Review,* reprinted in *The Living Age* 838, no. 23 (June 1860): 741.

17. Florence Nightingale, *Notes on Nursing: What It Is and What It Is Not,* first American edition (New York: D. Appleton and Company, 1860), 11.

18. Nightingale, *Notes on Nursing,* 87.

19. Ibid., 28, 41–42.

20. See the discussion in Judith Ann Giesburg, *Civil War Sisterhood: The U.S. Sanitary Commission and Women's Politics in Transition* (Boston: Northeastern University Press, 2000), 16–28.

21. The "handicraft" part of nursing should not, Nightingale acknowledged, be undervalued. "A patient," she admitted near the end of *Notes on Nursing,* "may be left bleed to death in a sanitary palace" (*Notes on Nursing,* 127).

22. Florence Nightingale, *Notes on Nursing for the Labouring Classes* (London: Harrison, 1861), 59.

23. Stuart Blumin, *The Emergence of the Middle Class: Social Experience in the American City* (New York: Cambridge University Press, 1989), 250–51.

24. D'Antonio, "Legacy of Domesticity."

25. See "To the Public, 1831," in "The Popularization of Voluntary Associations," 14, http://ksghome.harvard.edu/~phall/05.%20Blacks.pdf. See also "To the Honorable Senate and House of the Commonwealth of Pennsylvania, January 1832," ibid., 16–22, for the testimony of the African American community that although they comprised approximately 8 percent of the population, their community numbered only 4 percent of those using the city's almshouse or out-

door relief programs, and for testimony that, although the community paid $2,500 in taxes, they used only $2,000 in services.

26. Jacqueline Miller, "Wages of Blackness: African American Workers and the Meaning of Race during Philadelphia's Yellow Fever Epidemic," *Pennsylvania Magazine of History and Biography* 29, no. 2 (2005): 163–94.

27. Anne Summers, "The Mysterious Demise of Sarah Gamp: The Domiciliary Nurse and Her Detractors, 1830–1860," *Victorian Studies* 32 (1989).

28. See, for example, Louisa May Alcott, *Hospital Sketches* (1863; repr. New York: Garland Publishing, 1984).

29. Lisa Rosner, "Thistle on the Delaware: Edinburgh Medical Education and Philadelphia Practice, 1800–1825," *Social History of Medicine* 5 (1992): 19–40; Susan Reverby, *Ordered to Care: The Dilemma of American Nursing, 1850–1945* (New York: Cambridge University Press, 1987).

30. See, for examples, *Baltimore Patriot*, January 12, 1830; *Pittsfield Sun*, February 27, 1840, and March 19, 1843; *Philadelphia Inquirer*, November 16, 1860, available from American Historical Newspapers 1860–1900 at http://infoweb.newsbank.com.

31. *Baltimore Patriot*, March 31, 1830, ibid.

32. Jane Schultz, *Women at the Front: Hospital Workers in Civil War America* (Chapel Hill: University of North Carolina Press, 2004), 21–39.

33. Ibid., 36, 102, 35–36, 145–77. Middle-class women who had served as Civil War nurses sought government clerical careers. Working-class women sought factory positions in the industrializing economy. African American women remained effectively locked into domestic service.

34. John Harley Warner, *The Therapeutic Perspective: Medical Practice, Knowledge and Identity in America, 1820–1885* (Cambridge, MA: Harvard University Press, 1986).

35. Katherine Okuda Klein, "The Growth of Man-Midwifery in Philadelphia" (Ph.D. diss., University of California, Riverside, 2002). See also Roberta West, *A History of Nursing in Pennsylvania* (Harrisburg, PA: The Pennsylvania State Nurses Association, 1926), 610.

36. Joseph Warrington, *The Nurses Guide* (Philadelphia: Thomas Cowperthwait and Co., 1836), 12.

37. O'Brien, "All a Woman's Life Can Bring," 13. I am grateful to Joan Lynaugh for helping me think about this process as a trade.

38. J. S. Longshore, *The Principles and Practice of Nursing, or a Guide to the Inexperienced: Designed to Instruct the Nurse in the Principles of Her Profession, and to Assist the Inexperienced in Performing the Various Duties Pertaining to the Sick Room. Adapted to Families, Nurses, and Young Physicians* (Philadelphia: Merrihew and Thompson, 1842), n.p.

39. Thomas Longshore, A Sketch of the Life and Work of Joseph Longshore, 1893, Archives and Special Collections of Women in Medicine and Homeopathy, Drexel University College of Medicine, H-150.

40. Ann Preston, *Nursing the Sick and the Training of Nurses* (Philadelphia: King and Baird, 1863).

41. Steven J. Peitzman, *A New and Untried Course: Woman's Medical College and Medical College of Pennsylvania, 1850–1998* (New Brunswick, NJ: Rutgers University Press, 2000).

42. See Ellen S. More, *Restoring the Balance: Women Physicians and the Profession of Medicine, 1850–1995* (Cambridge, MA: Harvard University Press, 1999), and Regina Markell Morantz-Sanchez, *Sympathy and Science: Women Physicians in American Medicine* (New York: Oxford University Press, 1985).

43. Editorial, *New York Evangelist* 24 (1862): 32.

44. Thomas Longshore, A Sketch, n.p.

45. Minutes of the Board of Lady Managers, September 1872, Archives and Special Collections of Women in Medicine and Homeopathy, Drexel University College of Medicine.

46. Preston, *Nursing the Sick*, 1–3, 13.

47. Ibid., 7–8.

48. Minutes of the Board of Lady Managers, September 1864, Woman's Hospital, Archives and Special Collections of Women in Medicine and Homeopathy, Drexel University College of Medicine.

49. Warner, *Therapeutic Perspective*, 1–13.

50. Charles P. Putnam, "Training Schools for Nurses in America: Read at the Annual Meeting of the Association, 1874," p. 6, National Library of Medicine Historical Collections, MDNM9603101-B.

51. Charles Rosenberg, *The Care of Strangers: The Rise of America's Hospital System* (New York: Basic Books, 1987), 97–121

52. Samuel Gross, *Remarks on the Training of Nurses* (Philadelphia: Collins Printer, 1869), 4.

53. Ibid.

54. Ibid., 14, 5.

55. S. Weir Mitchell, "Nurse and Patient," *Lippincott's Magazine of Popular Literature and Science,* 10 (December 1872): 668, 669–76

56. Abram Livezy, Mothers' Department, *Peterson's Magazine* 72 (October 1877): 294. See also Livezy, Mothers' Department, *Peterson's Magazine* 62 (November 1872).

57. Frank Fisher, "The Trained Nurse," *Ladies Home Journal and Practical Housekeeper* 6 (April 1889): 4.

58. Philadelphia's *Friends' Intelligencer* (September 30, 1871), 489–91, reprinted parts of Hinton's popular *Thoughts on Health*.

59. W. G. Thompson, *Training Schools for Nurses with Notes on Twenty-Two Schools* (Philadelphia: G. P. Putnam's Sons, 1883), 8.

60. See Warner, *Therapeutic Perspective*, 241, and Rosenberg, *Care of Strangers*, 122–41.

61. See, for example, Anna Fullerton, *A Handbook of Obstetric Nursing, for Nurses, Students and Mothers; Comprising the Course of Instruction in Obstetric Nursing Given to the Pupils of the Training School for Nurses Connected with the Woman's Hospital of Philadelphia* (p. iv), National Library of Medicine, History of Medicine Division, WYF971h.

62. Clara S. Weeks, *A Textbook of Nursing for the Use of Training Schools, Families and Private Students* (New York: Appleton and Co., 1885), 21.

63. Elizabeth Gregg, "The Tuberculosis Nurse under Municipal Direction," *Public Health Nursing Quarterly* 5 (October 1913): 16.

64. James Wilson, *Fever Nursing; Designed for the Use of Professional and Other Nurses, and Especially as a Text-Book for Nurses in Training* (Philadelphia: J. B. Lippincott, 1888), 64.

65. John Eaton, *Circulars of Information of the Bureau of Education No.1-1879, Training Schools for Nurses* (Washington, DC: Government Printing Office, 1879), 5.

66. C. H. Crandall, "Amateur Classes in Nursing," *North American Review* 157, no. 445 (December 1893): 756–57.

67. "Amateur Nurses," *Littell's Living Age* 124, no. 1596 (1875): 125–27.

68. John Harley Warner, "Ideals of Science and Their Discontents in Late Nineteenth-Century American Medicine," *Isis*, 92 (1991): 455–78.

69. Horatio Storer, *Nurses and Nursing with Special Reference to the Management of Sick Women* (Boston: Lee and Shepard, 1868), 10.

70. Quoted in Dorothy Giles, *A Candle in Her Hands: A Story of the Nursing Schools of Bellevue Hospital* (New York: G. P. Putnam's Sons, 1945), 85–87.

71. John H. Packard, "Training of Nurses for the Sick: Read Before the Social Science Association of Philadelphia, June 1876," p. 10, College of Physicians of Philadelphia, PAM14513.

72. Boston Medical Library's Directory for Nurses 1879–1914, volume 1, editorial 10/24/1881: "Boston Trained Nurses in Chicago," in Countway Library, Harvard University, BMSb120.1.

73. See Kenneth Ludmerer, *Learning to Heal: The Development of American Medical Education* (New York: Basic Books, 1985), 13.

74. For information on Pauline Henry, see Notes and Queries, *Pennsylvania Magazine of History and Biography* 7 (1883): 108.

75. D'Antonio, "Legacy of Domesticity," 241.

76. The letters about these negotiation are reproduced in Roberta West, *Nursing in Pennsylvania*, 852–54.

77. Minutes of the Board of Lady Managers of the Woman's Hospital, January 1876 through October 1878, Archives and Special Collections of Women in Medicine and Homeopathy, Drexel University College of Medicine.

78. O'Brien, "All a Woman's Life Can Bring," 16.

79. Wilson, *Fever Nursing*, 39.

80. See Blumin, *Emergence of the Middle Class*, 66–107.

81. Agnes G. Deans and Anne L. Austin, *The History of the Farrand Training School for Nurses* (Detroit, MI: Alumnae Association of the Farrand Training School for Nurses, 1936), 35.

82. S. Weir Mitchell, *Address to the Graduating Class at the Annual Commencement of the Training School for Nurses of the Hospital of the University of Pennsylvania* (Philadelphia: John C. Winston Company, 1908), 11.

83. J. F. May, "Trained Nursing for the Home," *Pictorial Review* 8, no. 2 (1906): 109.

84. See, for example, "Nursing the Sick," in *Godey's Lady's Book and Magazine* 104 (February 1882): 620.

85. Carrie Niles Whitcomb, "Training Schools for Domestic Servants," *The Century: A Popular Quarterly* 52, no. 5 (1896): 796. See also Mrs. M.E.W. Sherwood, "The Lack of Good Servants," *North American Review* 153, no. 420 (1891): 546–59.

86. *A Handbook of Nursing for Families and General Use Published under the Direction of the Connecticut Training School for Nurses, State Hospital, New Haven, Connecticut* (Philadelphia: J. B. Lippincott, 1878), 10.

87. Alfred Stille, Address of the President, *Transactions of the American Medical Association* 12 (1871): 90.

88. *Historical Statistics of the United States*, Millennial Edition Online, Table Bd241–256.

Chapter Two: Competence, Coolness, Courage—and Control

1. Elizabeth Jones, "The Negro Woman in the Nursing Profession," *The Messenger* 5 (July 1923): 764.

2. Ibid., 765. Darlene Clark Hine, in "Black Professionals and Race Consciousness: Origins of the Civil Rights Movement, 1890–1950," *Journal of American History* 89, no. 4 (2003): 1279–94, addresses the role that professional physicians, lawyers, and nurses played in setting the stage for the later civil rights movement.

3. *Historical Statistics of the United States,* Millennial Edition Online, Series Bd241–256, Table 2-541.

4. Isabel Hampton Robb, "Educational Standards for Nurses," in *Educational Standards for Nurses and Other Addresses on Nursing Subjects* (Cleveland, OH: E. C. Koeckert, 1907), 15.

5. Charles Rosenberg, *The Care of Strangers: The Rise of America's Hospital System* (New York: Basic Books, 1987), 183.

6. See "Discussion on Caring for Male Patients," Annual Convention of the American Society of Superintendents of Training Schools for Nurses, 1896. Reprinted as *Annual Conventions 1893–1899: The American Society of Superintendents of Training Schools for Nurses* (New York: Garland Publishing, 1985), 70.

7. Jonathan Imber describes a similarly self-conscious approach to content and character among nineteenth-century physicians. See his *Trusting Doctors: The Decline of Moral Authority in American Medicine* (Princeton, NJ: Princeton University Press, 2008).

8. Barbara Miller Solomon, *In the Company of Educated Women: A History of Women and Higher Education in America* (New Haven, CT: Yale University Press, 1985), 44, 61, 64.

9. John R. Thelin, *A History of American Higher Education* (Baltimore: Johns Hopkins University Press, 2004), 169.

10. Solomon, *In the Company,* 63.

11. Ibid., 77.

12. Ibid., 61.

13. Amy Thompson McCandless, *Women's Higher Education in the Twentieth-Century American South* (Tuscaloosa: University of Alabama Press, 1999).

14. Solomon, *In the Company,* 145–56.

15. Ibid., 56–57.

16. S. Weir Mitchell, "Address to the Students of Radcliffe College, Delivered January 17, 1895," p. 6. Harvard University—Schlesinger Library on the History of Women in America, Open Collections Project: "Women Working, 1800–1930," http://ocp.hul.harvard.edu/ww/ .

17. Mitchell, "Address to the Graduating Class at the Annual Commencement of the Training School for Nurses of the Hospital of the University of Pennsylvania, November 24, 1908," pp. 5, 6. Harvard University—Schlesinger Library on the History of Women in America, Open Collections Project: "Women Working, 1800–1930," http://ocp.hul.harvard.edu/ww/.

18. Robb, "Nurse as Citizen," in *Educational Standards,* 264.

19. Nancy F. Noel, "Isabel Adams Hampton Robb, 1860–1910," in *American Nursing: A Biographical Dictionary,* ed. Vern L. Bullough, Olga M. Church, and Alice P. Stein (New York: Garland Publishing, 1988), 274–76.

20. Janet Wilson James, "Isabel Hampton and the Professionalizing of Nursing in the 1890s," in *Enduring Issues in American Nursing,* ed. Ellen D. Baer, Patricia D'Antonio, Sylvia Rinker, and Joan Lynaugh (New York: Springer Publishing, 2001), 45.

21. Isabel Hampton, "Educational Standards for Nurses," in *Hospitals, Dispensaries and Nursing,* ed. John S. Billings and Henry M. Hurd (repr., New York: Garland Publishing, 1984), 31, 33, 32.

22. June Schultz, *Nurses at the Front: Hospital Workers in Civil War America* (Chapel Hill: University of North Carolina Press, 2004), 119.

23. Hampton, "Educational Standards for Nurses," 32.

24. Historians Alison Bashford, Susan Reverby, and Kathryn McPherson have commented on the complex and sometimes contradictory ways in which nurses have historically used, created, and changed science. See Alison Bashford, "Domestic Scientists: Gender and the Negotiation of Science in Australian Nursing, 1880–1910," *Journal of Women's History* 12, no. 2 (2000); Susan Reverby, "A Legitimate Relationship: Nursing, Hospitals, and Science in the Twentieth Century," in *The American General Hospital: Communities and Social Contexts,* ed. Diana Elizabeth Long and Janet Golden (Ithaca, NY: Cornell University Press, 1989), 135–56; Kathryn McPherson, "Science and Technique: Nurses' Work in a Canadian Hospital, 1920–1939," in *Caring and Curing: Historical Perspectives on Women and Healing in Canada,* ed. Dianne Dodd and Deborah Gorham (Ottawa: University of Ottawa Press, 1994), 71–101.

25. Martha Lenora Collett Soper Lecture Notes, Barbara Bates Center for the Study of the History of Nursing, MC 61, folder 1, April 16, 1920.

26. Hamilton P. Jones, *Notes from Lectures Delivered Before The Training School for Nurses of the Charity Hospital* (New Orleans: J. G. Hauser, 1912), 80.

27. Cynthia Gurney, "Annie Warburton Goodrich," in *American Nursing,* 145–49.

28. Goodrich, "The Hospital and the Community, Read before the American Hospital Association, 1924," in Annie Warburton Goodrich, *The Social and Ethical Significance of Nursing* (New York: Macmillan, 1932), 150.

29. Goodrich, "The Need of Orientation, Read to the New York Academy of Medicine, 1912," in *Social and Ethical Significance,* 31.

30. As cited in Ellen S. More, *Restoring the Balance: Women Physicians and the Profession of Medicine, 1850–1995* (Cambridge, MA: Harvard University Press, 1999), 75.

31. Goodrich, "The Complete Nurse, Read Before the Metropolitan Training School, 1912," in *Social and Ethical Significance*, 41.

32. Goodrich, "Education and Training, published in *Modern Hospital*, 1921," in Goodrich, *Social and Ethical Significance*, 85.

33. 5th Annual Convention 1898, *Annual Conventions 1893-1899: The American Society of Superintendents of Training Schools for Nurses* (New York: Garland Publishing, 1985), 45.

34. Robb, "Nurse as Citizen," in *Educational Standards for Nurses*, 253-55.

35. Robb, "The Quality of Thoroughness in Nurses' Work," in *Educational Standards for Nurses*, 206-7.

36. 5th Annual Convention, "How are Training Schools Responsible for the Lack of Ethics among Nurses?" 45.

37. Editorial, *American Journal of Nursing* 17, no. 2 (1903): 101-102; "Alchemy of Influence, 1903," Philadelphia School of Nursing Medical Supply and Dispensary, Barbara Bates Center for the Study of the History of Nursing, AC box 1.

38. Stephanie Shaw, *What a Woman Ought to Be and Do: Black Professional Women Workers During the Jim Crow Era* (Chicago: University of Chicago Press, 1996).

39. Extract from a Probationer's Diary from the Orange, New Jersey Hospital Training School, www.aahn.org/trainingcirca1884.html.

40. Soper, Lecture Notes, 155-60.

41. For examples, see Lavinia Dock, *Materia Medica*, 3rd ed. (New York: G. P. Putnam's Sons, 1904); Emily Stoney, *Practical Materia Medica for Nurses with an Appendix*, 3rd ed. (Philadelphia: W. B. Saunders, 1912).

42. See, for example, Isabel Hampton Robb, *Nursing: Its Principles and Practices for Hospital and Private Use*, 2nd ed. (Cleveland: E. C. Koeckert, 1903), 484-500.

43. Byron Good, *Medicine, Rationality, and Experience: An Analytical Perspective* (New York: Cambridge University Press, 1994), 74.

44. Joan Lynaugh, "What We Know, We See," keynote address to the University College Dublin School of Nursing and Midwifery, March 2005.

45. See Goodrich, "The Complete Nurse," in *Social and Ethical Significance*, 42.

46. See Goodrich, "Social Service Course," in *Social and Ethical Significance*, 74.

47. Nell Elizabeth Peckens Pease Papers, Schlesinger Library, Radcliffe Institute for Advanced Study, 92-M170, box 1 (n.d., circa 1916).

48. (No author), "Culture and Training Schools," *American Journal of Nursing* 17, no. 12 (1917): 101–2.

49. Probationer's Diary, www.aahn.org/features/training2.html.

50. Robb, *Nursing*, 69.

51. Robert Baker, Arthur Caplan, Linda Emanuel, and Stephen Latham, eds., *The American Medical Ethics Revolution: How the AMA's Code of Ethics Has Transformed Physicians' Relationships to Patients, Professionals, and Society*, Appendix E, "Principles of Medical Ethics," 1912: 349–50, 351 (Baltimore: Johns Hopkins University Press, 1999).

52. Ibid., 351. Isabel Hampton Robb, *Nursing Ethics for Hospital and Private Use* (Cleveland: E. C. Koeckert, 1900), 98–104. See also Beth Linker, "The Business of Ethics: Gender, Medicine, and the Professional Codification of the American Physiotherapy Association, 1918–1935," *Journal of the History of Medicine and Allied Sciences* 60, no. 3 (2005): 320–54.

53. Mary Cadwalader Jones, "The Training of a Nurse," *Scribner's Magazine* 8, no. 5 (1890): 617.

54. Ibid., 615.

55. Anna Fullerton, *Surgical Nursing* (Philadelphia: P. Blakiston, Son & Co, 1891), 18.

56. Dock, "An Experiment in Contagious Nursing," 1903, in Janet James, ed., *Lavinia Dock Reader* (New York: Garland, 1985), 20.

57. Hamilton P. Jones, *Notes from Lectures*, 293.

58. Agnes Brennan, "Theory and Practice," Proceedings of the National Conference of Charities and Corrections, Nashville, Tennessee, 1894; reprinted in *Nurses Work: Issues Across Time and Place*, ed. Patricia D'Antonio, Ellen D. Baer, Sylvia Rinker, and Joan L. Lynaugh (New York: Springer Publishing, 2007), 289.

59. Maud Banfield, "The Journal's Trained Nurse Tells What to Do for Pneumonia," *Ladies Home Journal* 21, no. 2 (1904): 28.

60. See, e.g., Fullerton, *Obstetrics;* Jones, *Notes from Lectures;* Clara Weeks Shaw, *A Textbook of Nursing* (New York: D. Appleton & Co., 1889), 261–70.

61. See, for example, "Nurses and Nursing," *Medical and Surgical Reporter* 59, no. 10 (Sept. 8, 1888): 317–18. Nurses also repeated this rhetoric. See, for example, the multiple editions of Emily Stoney's *Practical Points for Nursing in Private Practice* (Philadelphia: W. B. Saunders, 1896 through 1911), xi.

62. See, for example, the obituary to Lilah Duncanson, a nursing supervisor who died of exposure to diphtheria, *Pacific Coast Journal of Nursing*, February 1920, 83. As Barbara Bates argues, a tuberculosis infection was almost a prerequisite for employment in a TB sanatorium. See *Bargaining for Life: A Social History of Tuberculosis, 1876–1935* (Philadelphia: University of Penn-

sylvania Press, 1992). Sarah C. Barry, from Providence Hospital in Rhode Island, surveyed her student and graduate nurses to see how many became sick after new techniques of aseptic nursing were introduced. In 1915 (the surveyed year) 1 graduate nurse of 46 (2%) and 19 student nurses of 353 (5%) contracted diphtheria. See "Aseptic Nursing of Infectious Diseases," *American Journal of Nursing* 16, no. 8 (1916): 687–92.

63. Jeanne Kisacky, "Restructuring Isolation: Hospital Architecture, Medicine, and Disease Prevention." *Bulletin of the History of Medicine* 79 (2005): 1–49.

64. D. L. Richardson, Aseptic Fever Nursing, *American Journal of Nursing* 15, no. 12 (1915): 1082–93 (quotes on 1083, 1084–85).

65. Minnie Goodnow, "Common Sense in Contagion," *Trained Nurse and Hospital Review* 54 (1915): 193–96, 270–72 (quote on 272). As cited in Kisacky's "Restructuring Isolation."

66. *Nursing Procedures at the Philadelphia General Hospital*, 1st ed., 1924: 116–118, Barbara Bates Center for the Study of the History of Nursing (BBCSHN).

67. See Bates, *Bargaining for Life*.

68. Goodrich, "Some Points of Weakness in Hospital Construction" in *Social and Ethical Significance*, 99.

69. Nellie S. Parks, "The Technic of Communicable Disease Nursing, *American Journal of Nursing* 22, no. 2 (1921): 81–82.

70. Sister Frieda, "A Combination Bassinet and Dressing Cabinet," *American Journal of Nursing* 32, no. 7 (1932): 746–48.

71. H. F. L. Locke, "Contact Theory of Transmission of Contagious Diseases," *American Journal of Nursing* 16, no. 11 (1916): 1093.

72. Robb, *Nursing*, 100.

73. George William Norris, Commencement Address to the Graduating Nurses of the Pennsylvania Hospital, April 10, 1913, Harvard University—Schlesinger Library on the History of Women in America, Open Collections Project: "Women Working, 1800–1930," http://ocp.hul.harvard.edu/ww/.

74. Yearbook of the Training School for Nurses at the Hospital for Sick Children, 1926. Children's Hospital School of Nursing Alumni Association Papers, 1906–1987, MSS 89-20, carton 1.

75. Regina Markell Morantz-Sanchez, *Sympathy and Science: Women Physicians in America* (New York: Oxford University Press, 1985), 254, 262.

76. Jennifer J. Fenne, "Every Woman Is a Nurse: Domestic Nursing in 19th-Century English Popular Literature" (Ph.D. diss., University of Wisconsin–Madison, 2000), 211.

77. Sara Wuthnow, "Our Mothers' Stories," *Nursing Outlook* 38 (1990): 221.

78. Lynda Anderson, "Report of the 15th Annual ANA Convention, *Pacific Coast Journal of Nursing*, August 1912, 371.

79. T. Gaillard Thomas, "Address to the Graduates of the Training School for Nurses of the Colored Home and Hospital," *Medical News,* February 15, 1902, 291 (retrieved from APS Online). See also George Norris, "Commencement Address to the Graduating Nurses of the Pennsylvania Hospital, April 10, 1913, Harvard University—Schlesinger Library on the History of Women in America, Open Collections Project: "Women Working, 1800–1930," http://ocp.hul .harvard.edu/ww/.

80. Lavinia Dock, "Ethics or a Code of Ethics," in James, *Lavinia Dock Reader,* 39.

81. John Harley Warner, *The Therapeutic Perspective: Medical Practice, Knowledge and Identity in America, 1820–1885* (Cambridge, MA: Harvard University Press, 1986), 65.

82. Thomas, "Address to the Graduates," 290.

83. Charles V. Chapin, 1913, "Address by Charles V. Chapin Delivered at the Graduating Exercises of the Butler Hospital Training School for Nurses, November 12, 1912" (Providence, RI: Snow and Farnham). See also Alfred Worcester's "Possibilities of a School of Nursing in Cambridge" (Read before the Cambridge Medical Improvement Society, October 24, 1904, Relative to the Cambridge School of Nursing, before the Cambridge Medical Improvement Society, the Colonial Club of Cambridge, and the Students of Radcliffe College), Harvard University—Schlesinger Library on the History of Women in America, Open Collections Project: "Women Working, 1800–1930," http://ocp.hul .harvard.edu/ww/. "Too often," Worcester noted, nurses "pity the common ordinary family doctor, whose methods of practice are so unlike those of the brilliant hospital physicians and surgeons under whom alone they have worked during their studentship" (5).

84. Mayme Williamson, "Advice to Nurses," *Pacific Coast Journal of Nursing,* August 1921, 48.

85. Susan Reverby, *Ordered to Care: The Dilemma of American Nursing, 1850–1945* (New York: Cambridge University Press, 1987), 97–98.

Chapter Three: They Went Nursing—in Early Twentieth-Century America

1. Corinne Johnson Kern, *I Go Nursing* (New York: E. P. Dutton & Co., 1933), 19, 21. This book proved so popular among lay audiences that she wrote two similar books for E. P. Dutton: *I Was a Probationer* (1937) and *Nursing through the Years* (1940).

2. Ibid., 16, 35, 81.

3. Ibid., 73,141, 144–46, 75.

4. Ibid., 57, 174, 108, 117.

5. See also the experiences recounted by Daisy Barnwell Jones in her memoir, *My First 80 Years* (Baltimore: Gateway Press, 1986).

6. Mary L. White, "The Training School for Nurses in San Francisco," *Overland Monthly and Out West Magazine*, February 1887, 123.

7. Gray Brechin, *Imperial San Francisco: Urban Power, Earthly Ruin* (Berkeley: University of California Press, 1999).

8. White, "Training School," 123.

9. Ibid., 123, 126.

10. For a history of the hospital, see Rickey Hendricks, "Feminism and Maternalism in Early Hospitals for Children: San Francisco and Denver, 1875–1915," *Journal of the West*, July 1993, 61–62.

11. M. A. Burrell Diary, UCSF Archives and Special Collections, MSS 81-1, 31 May 1900. Burrell's diary indicated that she was born in 1856, so she would have been much older than most training school students. For a brief description of the 1st Reserve Hospital, see J.D.M.'s "Experiences in Army Nursing," *American Journal of Nursing* 3 (September 1903): 948–49.

12. Burrell Diary, September 1900 (n.d.), June 1900 (n.d.), December 1904 (n.d.).

13. Burrell Diary, 8 October 1904–3 December 1904, 3 December 1904, 9 November 1912, 27 July 1913, 1914 (n.d.), 18 May–1 June 1915.

14. Eugenia Venegas, "Three Nurses and a Chicken Ranch," *Overland Monthly and Out West Magazine* 44, no. 3 (1904), retrieved from APS Online, pp. 0–011.

15. For examples across the country, see Children's Hospital, UCSF Archives and Special Collections, Children's Hospital School of Nursing Alumni Association Papers, 1906–1987, MSS 89-20, carton 1. For the Hospital of the University of Pennsylvania, see "The Directory of Graduates of the School of Nursing of the Hospital of the University of Pennsylvania," 8–11, Barbara Bates Center for the Study of the History of Nursing. For Farrand, see Agnes Deans and Anne L. Austin, *The History of the Farrand Training School for Nurses* (Detroit, MI: Alumnae Association of the Farrand Training School for Nurses, 1938), 161.

16. Burrell Diary, 6 June 1904.

17. Ibid., 1 August–3 August 1915.

18. Lucy Wimbash to "Mother," March 8, 1908, Wimbash Family Collection, 1852–1939, University of Virginia Small Collections, #8979-v-w.

19. Emitt Wimbash to "my precious mammy," August 20, 1908.

20. *History of St. Luke's Hospital Training School for Nurses, May 1888–May 1938* (privately printed, 1938), 9–38. I am grateful to Jean Whelan for giving me this resource.

21. Ibid., 9–65; 62, 78. From 1918 to 1934, St. Luke's charged its students an entrance fee of $25. This fee was raised to $50 in 1934.

22. Data was compiled from the careers of every fifth graduate of each graduating class listed in the Appendix to *History of St. Luke's.*

23. See UCSF Archives and Special Collections, Children's Hospital School of Nursing Alumni Association Papers, 1906–1987, MSS 89-20, carton 1. Sixty-three percent of graduates of the Children's Hospital Training School Class of 1896 remained single as did 67 percent of all graduates between 1890 and 1899.

24. *History of St. Luke's,* 177, 218, 177.

25. Nancy Tomes also found this pattern in her study of the Pennsylvania Hospital Training School for Nurses in Philadelphia. See Tomes, "'A Little World of Our Own': The Pennsylvania Hospital Training School for Nurses, 1895–1907," in *Women and Health in America: Historical Readings,* ed. Judith Leavitt (Madison: University of Wisconsin Press, 1984).

26. *History of St. Luke's,* 258, 121, 216. Stoddart maintained an interest in health and hospital work throughout her married life; she remained active as a volunteer for her local Red Cross chapter and at her local hospital. Reverby found similar movement between positions among Massachusetts nurses in her *Ordered to Care: The Dilemma of American Nursing, 1850–1945* (New York: Cambridge University Press, 1987), 111–18.

27. Adelaide Brown, "The Outlook for a Graduate Nurse," 1924, UCSF Archives and Special Collections, MSS 89-20, series IV, box 1 OS.

28. *History of St. Luke's,* 137, 307. See also the careers of Mabel Gould Carver (1919), Anstisse Bishop (1915), and Elsa Zeller (1914), in ibid., 86, 105, 273.

29. See Charles Rosenberg, *The Care of Strangers: The Rise of America's Hospital System* (New York: Basic Books, 1987), 310–20.

30. *History of St. Luke's,* 301–2.

31. Ibid., 59. St. Luke's data remain silent on the issue that one factor pushing nurses out of social service roles may have been the development of the field of social work. See Daniel Walkowitz, *Working with Class: Social Workers and the Politics of Middle Class Identity* (Chapel Hill: University of North Carolina Press, 1999).

32. Ibid., 59.

33. Yssabella Waters, *Visiting Nursing in the United States* (New York: Charities Committee Publication, 1909), 86.

34. For the history of public health nursing, see Karen Buhler-Wilkerson's *False Dawn: The Rise and Fall of Public Health Nursing in America* (New York: Garland Press, 1983), and her *No Place Like Home: A History of Nursing and Home Care in the United States* (Baltimore: Johns Hopkins University Press, 2001). See also Diane Hamilton, "The Cost of Caring: The Metropolitan Life Insurance Company's Visiting Nurse Service, 1909–1953," *Bulletin of the History of Medicine* 63, no. 3 (1989): 414–34.

35. *History of St. Luke's*, 246–47.

36. Children's Hospital Alumni Association Papers, 1906–1987, MSS 89-20, carton 1.

37. Buhler-Wilkerson, *False Dawn*, 98.

38. See Peggy Pascoe, *Relations of Rescue: The Search for Female Moral Authority in the American West, 1874–1939* (New York: Oxford University Press, 1990).

39. See Jane Hitchcock, "Visiting Nursing: Report of the Sub-Committee," *American Journal of Nursing* 6, no. 1 (1905): 26–29.

40. Yssabella Waters, *Visiting Nursing in the United States* (New York: Charities Committee Publication, 1909), 45–49 and 86–123. For more information on public health nursing in California, see Octavia Briggs, "Tehama Street Settlement," *Journal of the California Nurses Association* 1, no. 1 (1904): 14–16.

41. "Public Health Nursing Report," *Pacific Coast Journal of Nursing*, November 1916, 685.

42. Sophia Balch, "A Day's Work in Public Health Nursing," *Pacific Coast Journal of Nursing*, May 1921, 295.

43. "Big Gift to Advance the Training of Nurses," *New York Times*, 3 December 1909. See also Beatrice and Philip Kalish, *The Advance of American Nursing*, 3rd ed. (Philadelphia: J. B. Lippincott, 1995), 196.

44. "Stanford University School of Nursing," *Pacific Coast Journal of Nursing*, November 1920, 686.

45. "Announcement," *Pacific Coast Journal of Nursing*, May 1921, 297. Another option for higher education for public health nurses lay in women's colleges such as Simmons in Boston, Massachusetts, which offered a certificate in public health.

46. Isabel Glover Bachels (autobiography), Bancroft Library, University of California, Berkeley, MSS 87/70, folders 3 and 4 (no pagination).

47. Ibid., folder 4

48. Ibid., folder 5 and folder 1.

49. The influenza pandemic did not strike Camp Logan as severely as it struck other military camps.

50. See Audrey Davis, "Edna Lois Foley," in *American Nursing: A Biographical Dictionary,* ed. Vern L. Bullough, Olga M. Church, and Alice P. Stein (New York: Garland Publishing, 1988), 115–17.

51. Bachels (autobiography), folder 5

52. See, for example, Steven J. Hoffman, "Progressive Public Health Administration in the Jim Crow South: A Case Study of Richmond, Virginia, 1907–1920, *Journal of Social History* 35, no. 1 (2001): 175–94; Marie Pitts Mosley, "Satisfied to Carry the Bag: Three Black Community Health Nurses' Contributions to Health Care Reform," *Nursing History Review* 4 (1996): 65–82; and Karen Buhler-Wilkerson, "Caring in its Proper Place: Race and Benevolence in Charleston, South Carolina, 1813–1939," *Nursing Research* 41, no. 1 (1992): 14–20.

53. Bachels (autobiography), folder 5.

54. Ibid., folder 6 and folder 7.

55. Ibid, folder 7.

56. Ibid, folder 7. Echoes of these same characteristics of a successful public health nurse appear in the novels of Mary Sewall Gardner, *So Build We* (1942) and *Katherine Kent* (1946). Gardner, another leader of early twentieth-century public health nursing, retired as the director of the Providence (Rhode Island) District Nurses Association in 1931. See Lois Monteiro's "Insights from the Past," *Nursing Outlook* 35 (1987): 65–69.

57. Bachels (autobiography), folder 8.

58. Many nurses who specialized in tuberculosis case finding and health teaching had, like Glover, had tuberculosis themselves. See Barbara Bates, *Bargaining for Life: A Social History of Tuberculosis, 1876–1935* (Philadelphia: University of Pennsylvania Press, 1992).

59. Bachels (autobiography), folder 1, folder 9, and folder 10

60. See Daisy Barnwell Jones, *My First Eighty Years.*

61. Bachels (autobiography), folder 10.

62. For a description of the nursing and medical staff arrangements, see Ethel Johns' "A Study of the Present State of the Negro Woman in Nursing," a Rockefeller Foundation study conducted in 1925 (typescript), Rockefeller Foundation Archives, Sleepy Hollow, New York, Exhibit A, 2–8.

63. Darlene Clark Hine, *Black Women in White: Racial Conflict and Cooperation in the Nursing Profession, 1890–1950* (Bloomington: Indiana University Press, 1989), 41–43.

64. Department of Nursing Education, Teachers' College, Columbia University, "A Survey of the Lincoln School for Nurses, New York City 1931" (typescript), Barbara Bates Center for the Study of the History of Nursing, 3, 152–61.

65. Ibid., 91–92, 5.

66. Ibid., 126.

67. See "Mary E. P. Mahoney (colored)," Boston Medical Library's Directory for Nurses, vol. 1, p. 114, Countway Library Center for the History of Medicine, Boston, Massachusetts. Mahoney was one of the founders of the National Association for Colored Graduate Nurses (NACGN) in 1908 and had a successful career until her retirement in 1912 at the age of 67 (see Althea Davis, "Mary Elizabeth Mahoney," in *American Nursing*, 226–27). Mahoney's life, like those of many other single women, became much more difficult after retirement. She depended on a pension from the Doane Fund, established by the white women who supported the nurses in Boston's Home for Aged Women, and a small stipend from the NACGN (Minutes of the NACGN, November 11, 1919, p. 81, Schomberg Center for Black Research and Culture, New York Public Library).

68. "Marguerite Harris Papers and Artifacts," Foundation of the New York State Nurses, Bellevue Alumnae Center for Nursing History, MC 10.

69. Althea Davis, "Adah Belle Samuels Thoms," in *American Nursing*, 313–16; Althea Davis, "Martha Minerva Franklin," in *American Nursing*, 120–23. For Hulda Margaret Lyttle, see www.answers.com/topic/hulda-margaret-lyttle.

70. Teacher's College, *Survey*, chap. 13, p. 163.

71. George Hutchinson, *In Search of Nella Larsen: A Biography of the Color Line* (Cambridge, MA: Belknap Press of Harvard University, 2006), 75. Much of the biographical material here comes from Hutchinson's work. See also Thadious Davis, *Nella Larsen, Novelist of the Harlem Renaissance: A Woman's Life Unveiled* (Baton Rouge: Louisiana State University Press, 1994).

72. Hutchinson, *In Search of Nella Larsen*, 463–65.

Chapter Four: Wives, Mothers—and Nurses

1. LDS School of Nursing Papers, L. Tom Perry Special Collections (LTPSC), Brigham Young University (BYU), UA 1020, box 7, vol. 1.

2. Additional biographical information can be found in the Maria Johnson Papers, LTPSC, BYU, MSS SC 371, folder 2.

3. Johnson Papers, MSS SC 371, folder 1.

4. *Utah Nurse* 4 (November–December 1950): 3.

5. For more current analyses, see John Mihelich and Debbie Storrs, "Higher Education and the Negotiated Process of Hegemony: The Embedded Resistance among Mormon Women," *Gender and Society* 17, no. 3 (2003): 404–22; Peggy Fletcher Stack, "Mormonism and Feminism?" *Wilson Quarterly* 15, no. 2 (1991): 30–32; Laurence Iannaccone and Carrie Miles, "Dealing with Social

Change: The Mormon Church's Response to Changes in Women's Roles," *Social Forces* 68 (1990): 1231–51.

6. See Carrel Hilton Sheldon, "Mormon Haters," in *Mormon Sisters: Women in Early Utah*, ed. Claudia L. Bushman (Logan: Utah State University Press, 1997), 113–32.

7. Thomas Alexander, *Utah: The Right Place*, 2nd rev. ed. (Salt Lake City: Gibbs, Smith Publishers, 2003), 126–55.

8. As cited in Claudia Lauper Bushman and Richard Lyman Bushman, *Mormons in America* (New York: Oxford University Press, 1999), 67.

9. For a discussion of early Mormon history and theology, see Bushman and Bushman, *Mormons in America*.

10. Jill Mulvey Derr, Janath Russell Cannon, and Maureen Ursenbach Beecher, *Women of Covenant: The Story of the Relief Society* (Salt Lake City: Deseret Book Company, 1992), x.

11. Bushman and Bushman, *Mormons in America*, 67.

12. Alexander, *Utah*, 154–75.

13. Thomas Alexander, *Mormonism in Transition: A History of Latter-day Saints, 1890–1930* (Urbana: University of Illinois Press, 1986), 14.

14. Alexander, *Mormonism in Transition*, 23–30.

15. Derr, Cannon, and Beecher, *Women of Covenant*, 151–79.

16. See Vella Neil Evan, "Mormon Women and the Right to Work," *Dialogue: The Journal of Mormon Thought* 23, no. 4 (1990): 46–61. See also Evan, "The Girl Who Earns Money," *Young Woman's Journal* 6 (1905): 490.

17. Circular letter to the leadership of the Relief Society from the 1st Presidency, 31 October 1914. LDS Church Archives, CR 11 8.

18. Lester E. Bush, *Health and Medicine among the Latter-day Saints* (New York: Crossroad, 1993), 88.

19. Alexander, *Utah*, 198, 218–49; and Alexander, *Mormons and Gentiles*, 2–13.

20. 1870 census data from Alexander, *Mormons and Gentiles*, 16–17; 1890 census data from the 13th Census of the United States (1910): Abstract (Washington, DC: Government Printing Office, 1913).

21. 13th Census of the United States (1910).

22. Alexander, *Mormons and Gentiles*.

23. Ibid., 109–12.

24. For details, see "St. Mark's Hospital School of Nursing," University of Utah Archives (UUA) RT80 U82 S33; and "A History of the Holy Cross Hospital School of Nursing," UUA, #588. For a more substantive treatment of the Holy Cross Hospital and its nuns, see Barbra Mann Wall, *Unlikely Entrepreneurs:*

Catholic Sisters and the Hospital Marketplace, 1865–1925 (Columbus: Ohio State University Press, 2005).

25. Alexander, *Utah*, 164.

26. Bush, *Health and Medicine*, 94–95.

27. Derr, Cannon, and Beecher, *Women of Covenant*.

28. *Salt Lake Sanitarian* 2, no. 1 (1889): 49, 141–42.

29. *Salt Lake Sanitarian* 1, no. 1 (1888): 27.

30. *Salt Lake Sanitarian* 2, no. 8 (1889): 49. See also Elaine Shaw Sorensen, "'For Zion's Sake': The Emergence of Mormon Nursing," *Nursing History Review* 6 (1998): 51–70.

31. *Salt Lake Sanitarian* 2, no. 8 (1889): 49.

32. Circular letters from Amy Brown Lyman, 17 August 1916 and 10 July 1917, LDS Church Archives, CR 11 8.

33. Sorenson, "For Zion's Sake," 51–70

34. Circular letter from the 1st President, 12 September 1918, LDS Church Archives, CR 11 8.

35. Hospital-based training was discontinued in 1924 when the program was not accredited by the New York State Board of Regents National Hospital Training School Rating Bureau, the certification and registration body officially recognized by the state of Utah (see Sorenson, "For Zion's Sake," 61).

36. For graduation lists, see *Relief Society Magazine* 4, no. 8 (1917): 453; 5, no. 7 (1918): 415–16; and 7, no. 7 (1920): 387–88.

37. Relief Society, box 1, folder 4, LDS Church Archives, CR 11 8.

38. "Graduation Exercises of the Relief Society Nurse Class," *Relief Society Magazine* 8, no. 10 (1921): 559; and "LDS Relief Society for Training Nurses Aids," *Relief Society Magazine* 7, no. 7 (1920), n.p.

39. See Susan Reverby, *Ordered to Care: The Dilemma of American Nursing, 1850–1945* (New York: Cambridge University Press, 1987), 77–94, for the best discussion of this crisis.

40. The exclusively female Army Nurse Corps had been created in 1901. See Mary Sarnecky, *A History of the U.S. Army Nurse Corps* (Philadelphia: University of Pennsylvania Press, 1999).

41. Reverby, *Ordered to Care*, 96–99.

42. In 1921, for example, new LDS Hospital student nurses had to bring $19 for uniforms and supplies. "History of the LDS Hospital School of Nursing, 1905–1955," LDS SON Alumnae Association Records, UA 1020, LTPSC, BYU, box 5, folder 4 (hereafter History of the LDS Hospital SON).

43. Alexander, *Utah*, 189–91.

44. For details, see John M. Barry's *The Great Influenza: The Epic Story of the Deadliest Plague in History* (New York: Viking, 2004), 341.

45. See Biography of Violet Larssen Olpin, LDS Church Archives, MS 17215.

46. These included the Dee Hospital in Ogden, Utah, and the Budge Hospital in Logan, Utah. See Robert T. Divitt, *Medicine and the Mormons: A History of the Latter-day Saints Health Care* (Bountiful, UT: Horizons Publishers, 1981).

47. History of the LDS Hospital SON, 54–55.

48. Ibid., 19, 38, 20.

49. Ibid., 36.

50. School admission ledgers that would contain letters of application no longer exist.

51. History of the LDS Hospital SON, 20, 22, 19.

52. Ibid., 49, 73.

53. 1965 *Facts About Nursing* (New York: National League for Nursing, 1966), 88. For data on collegiate education and white women in 1952, the most comparable year for which statistics are available, see U.S. Census Bureau statistics at www.census.gov/population/socdemo/education/tableA-2.txt, released 19 December 2000. Not all degrees were in nursing for nursing careers.

54. For early biographical information, see www.geocities.com/hillypippin/manuscript.pdf; for Newark VNA data, see http://digital.lib.usa.edu; for USU data, see personal correspondence with Bob Parson, archivist, 31 January 2006.

55. Yancy had seven children and died in childbirth. See History of the LDS Hospital SON, 37, and Yancey Ancestral File Notes (AFN): 5LZN-NL, Family History Library, Church of Jesus Christ of Latter-day Saints, Salt Lake City, Utah. Access to AFN is also available through www.familysearch.org/Eng/default.asp.

56. History of the LDS Hospital SON, 37. Thatcher Shaw AFN: 2S6V-T7, Family History Library, Church of Jesus Christ of Latter-day Saints, Salt Lake City, Utah.

57. Kathryn McPherson, *Bedside Matters: The Transformation of Canadian Nursing, 1900–1990* (Oxford: Oxford University Press, 1996).

58. History of the LDS Hospital SON, 60.

59. Ibid., 37.

60. Ibid., 19–20.

61. This represents an ever-married rate compiled from data from the classes of 1908, 1910, 1912, 1914, 1916, 1918, 1919, 1920, 1922, and 1924. See also Alumnae Association Minutes, 15 February 1926 and 26 October 1926. LTPSC BYU LDS School of Nursing Alumni Records, 1908–1985, UA 1020 box 1, folder 1.

62. May Ayres Burgess, *Nurses, Patients, and Pocketbooks: A Study of the Economics of Nursing by the Committee on the Grading of Training Schools* (New York: Committee on the Grading of Nursing Schools, 1928), 53–54.

63. See Helga Kruger and Bernd Baldus, "Work, Gender and the Life Course: Social Construction and Individual Experience," *Canadian Journal of Sociology* 23, no. 3 (1999): 355–79, for current sociological analyses of how aggregate data often hide significant discontinuities in women's work experiences that challenge assumptions of "normal" life-cycle work paths.

64. Lee L. Bean, Geraldine Mineau, and Douglas Anderton, *Fertility Change on the American Frontier: Adaptation and Innovation* (Berkeley: University of California, 1990). See also Ann S. Lee, "Interstate Differences in Fertility in the United States, 1910–1960" (Ph.D. diss., University of Pennsylvania, 1996).

65. See, for example, the essays in *Women's Position and Demographic Change*, ed. Nora Federici, Karen Oppenheim Mason, and Sølvi Sogner (Oxford: Clarendon Press, 1993).

66. Mary Powell Lindsay Papers, LTPSC BYU SC 1044.

67. Christine Bose, *Women in 1900: Gateway to the Political Economy of the Twentieth Century* (Philadelphia: Temple University Press, 2001).

68. See Burton Bledstein and Robert D. Johnson, eds., *The Middling Sorts: Explorations in the History of the American Middle Class* (New York and London: Routledge, 2001).

69. History of the LDS Hospital SON, 40.

70. "Biography, reminiscences, and concise genealogy and posterity of Violet Larsson Olpin 2001," LDS Church Archives, MS 17215.

71. *A History of the Holy Cross School of Nursing*, UUA, Accn 588, p. 56.

72. History of the LDS Hospital SON, 36–40.

73. Ibid., 36–41. Certainly, this number may well mask the numbers of 1919 graduates employed in family businesses, on farms, or in other home-based income-generating strategies such as boarding or laundry.

74. Ruth Partridge, *Adventures with a Lamp: The Story of a Nurse* (New York: Dutton, 1939).

75. Biography of Amelia Latta, LDS Church History Archives, MS D 2735 223.

76. History of the LDS Hospital SON, 20.

77. See, for example, Susan Porter Benson, *Counter Cultures: Saleswomen, Managers, and Customers in American Department Stores, 1890–1949* (Urbana: University of Illinois Press, 1986); Eileen Boris, *Home to Work: Motherhood and the Politics of Industrial Homework in the United States* (New York: Cambridge University Press, 1994); Bose, *Women in 1900;* and Joanne

Meyerowitz, *Women Adrift: Independent Wage Earners in Chicago, 1880–1930* (Chicago: University of Chicago Press, 1998).

78. The Freedmen's Hospital itself had opened in 1863 to care for sick southern African Americans flocking into the city during the Civil War. The training school had opened in 1894 with a white nursing superintendent. But in 1921 Emma Irwin, an African American graduate of Provident Hospital Training School for Nurses in Chicago, had assumed control. See *The Freedmen's Hospital School of Nursing, 1894–1973* (Washington, DC: Freedmen Hospital School of Nursing, 1973), 7–9. One white observer, in a 1923 visit to the school, was impressed. The school itself was, in her opinion, "the best developed training school for nurses under colored direction," and Irwin, she reported, was widely regarded among both her African American and her white supporters as a woman of "considerable ability and vision." See Ethel Johns, "A Study of the Present Status of the Negro Woman in Nursing" (typescript), Rockefeller Foundation Archives, Sleepy Hollow, New York, G-3.

79. "Irene Scott Williams," *The Fifty Year Graduates of the Freedmen's Hospital School of Nursing Tell Their Story* (Washington, DC: Freedmen's Hospital Nurses Alumni Clubs, Inc., 1986), 27. Barbara Bates Center for the Study of the History of Nursing, MC 25, folder 5.

80. "Aileen Cole Steward," *Fifty Year Graduates*, 37.

81. Ibid., 35.

Chapter Five: Race, Place, and Professional Identity

1. Jacqueline C. Zalumas, "Jane Van de Vrede," in *American Nursing: A Biographical Dictionary*, ed. Vern L. Bullough, Olga M. Church, and Alice P. Stein (New York: Garland Publishing, 1988), 333–36.

2. Adelaide Nutting, "Suggestions for the Educational Standards for State Registration, Delivered to the International Council of Nurses in 1904," in *A Sound Economic Basis for Schools of Nursing and Other Addresses* (repr., New York: Garland Press, 1984), 62. National nursing leaders were careful to admit that it was "occasionally" possible to provide a good nursing education in a small institution. See the late-1920s canvas of American training schools, in "The Second Grading of Nursing Schools," p. 9, Barbara Bates Center for the Study of the History of Nursing.

3. Susan Reverby, *Ordered to Care: The Dilemma of American Nursing, 1850–1945* (New York: Cambridge University Press, 1987), 160–64 (for "passing," see 163). Karen Buhler-Wilkerson, *False Dawn: The Rise and Fall of Public Health Nursing in America* (New York: Garland Press, 1983), 89–106.

4. ANA Southern Division Records #4759, Southern Historical Collection, University of North Carolina, Chapel Hill, box 1, folder 1. Van de Vrede was a consistently supporter of African American nursing ambitions. See Carla Schissel, "The State Nurses' Association in a Georgia Context" (Ph.D. diss., Emory University, 1979), 248.

5. See, for example, Marjorie Stimson and Louise Tattershall, "A Study of Negro Public Health Nursing," *Public Health Nurse*, October 1930, 532. See also Linda Sabin, "Unheralded Nurses: Male Caregivers in the 19th Century South," *Nursing History Review* 5 (1997): 31–48, for her argument that high-status white men held a place within southern nursing traditions during epidemics and disasters.

6. See http://historymatters.gmu.edu/d/39/.

7. For an overview, see C. Vann Woodward, *Origins of the New South, 1877–1913* (Baton Rouge: Louisiana State University Press, 1951); William A. Link, *The Paradox of Southern Progressivism, 1880–1930* (Chapel Hill: University of North Carolina Press, 1992).

8. See Gregory Mixon, *The Atlanta Race Riot: Race, Class and Violence in a New Southern City* (Gainesville: University Press of Florida, 2005).

9. Ethel Johns, "A Study of the Present Status of the Negro Woman in Nursing," unpublished manuscript, Rockefeller Foundation Archives, Sleepy Hollow, New York, Appendix G, p. 8.

10. Georgia Hickey, *Hope and Danger in the New South City: Working Class Women and Urban Development in Atlanta, 1890–1940* (Athens: University of Georgia Press, 2003).

11. Margaret Ellen Kidd Parsons, "White Plague and Double Barred Cross in Atlanta, 1895–1945" (Ph.D. diss., Emory University, 1985).

12. As quoted in ibid., 63.

13. The most detailed examination of the role of these women's associations within hospitals can be found in Jane Mottus, *New York Nightingales: The Emergence of the Nursing Profession at Bellevue and New York Hospital, 1850–1920* (Ann Arbor: University of Michigan Research Press, 1980), 23–62.

14. Grady Hospital Auxiliary Archives, Georgia State Archives, DOC 5816, folder 1, September 1894 to October 1894.

15. Ibid., March 1895.

16. Ibid., January 1896. Grady also refused requests from smaller hospitals for affiliation requests (see Minutes of the Medical Board, Grady Memorial Hospital Collection, Atlanta History Center, box 3, October 14, 1913). For information on Spelman, see www.georgiaencyclopedia.org/nge/Article.jsp?id=h-1460.

17. Grady Hospital Auxiliary Archives, September 1898 through August 1899. The Grady Hospital Training School eventually opened a nurses' home for white students in 1918 after it received a private donation. See Grady Hospital Training School Bulletin, 1918, at the Auburn Avenue Research Library on African American Culture and History, Atlanta-Fulton Public Library System, National Grady Nurses Conclave, box 7.

18. Minutes of the Medical Board, June 11, 1907.

19. Ibid., April 11, 1911.

20. Ibid., 1911 Report of the Committee on Medical Matters to the Medical Board.

21. Ibid., March 18, 1910.

22. Ibid., April 11, 1911.

23. Hickey, *Hope and Danger*, 44, points out that changing jobs was one of the most effective strategies white working southern women used to control their work experience. She uses the example of nurse Annie Alexander, who changed jobs so that she "could always get to Church on Sunday."

24. Minutes of the Medical Board, Report of the Medical Committee, December 9, 1913, and April 8, 1913.

25. Minutes of the Medical Board, December 9, 1913

26. Ibid., February 3, 1916, and November 11, 1919. By 1919, after two years of military nursing service in World War I, Feebeck returned to Grady. Her reputation now was such that she was immediately recruited by the Georgia Baptist Hospital to run its training school. Grady convinced Feebeck to stay with a substantive salary increase.

27. Ibid., June 9, 1912.

28. For the white medical board perspective, see Minutes of the Medical Board, October 10, 1914. For Andrews' perspective, see "The Beginning," and Appendix D (letter from Ludie Andrews to Mrs. Kemper Harrold, February 24, 1926) in Verdelle B. Bellamy, ed., *The History of Grady Memorial Hospital School of Nursing*, n.p., National Grady Nurses Conclave, Auburn Avenue Research Library on African American Culture and History, Atlanta-Fulton Public Library System, box 7.

29. Minutes of the Medical Board, October 10, 1914; September 12, 1916.

30. This prestige and exclusiveness, as historians have long pointed out, served as a proxy for white, middle-class privilege. See Nancy Tomes, "The Silent Battle: Nurse Registration in New York State, 1903–1920," in *Nursing History: New Perspectives, New Possibilities*, ed. Ellen Lagemann (New York: Teachers College Press, 1983), 107–32; Susan Armeny, "Resolute Enthusiasts: The Effort to Professionalize American Nursing, 1880–1915"

(Ph.D. diss., University of Missouri–Columbia, 1985); and Reverby, *Ordered to Care.*

31. For another examination of Andrews' battle, see Darlene Clark Hine, *Black Women in White: Racial Conflict and Cooperation in the Nursing Profession, 1890–1950* (Bloomington: Indiana University Press, 1989), xx–xxi, 93.

32. Schissel, "State Nurses' Association," 238–66.

33. Ibid., 244.

34. See newspaper clippings and historical sketches from the 1950s and 60s in Bellamy, *History of Grady Memorial Hospital School of Nursing.*

35. It remains unclear why the GSNA capitulated in 1919. It is probable that the association, looking at the experiences of its southern neighbors, realized that the registration of African American nurses did not breach the color line because training experiences and employment remained strictly segregated..

36. "Dorothy Banfield," box 1, and "Helen Smith," box 3, Georgia Public Health Nurses Oral History Collection, MSS #733, Manuscript, Archives, and Rare Book Library, Emory University (hereafter Georgia Oral History Collection).

37. May Ayres Burgess, *Nurses, Patients, and Pocketbooks: A Study of the Economics of Nursing by the Committee on the Grading of Nursing Schools* (New York: Committee on the Grading of Training Schools, 1928), 103.

38. James O. Breeden, "Disease as a Factor in Southern Distinctiveness," in *Disease and Distinctiveness in the American South,* ed. Todd Savitt and James Harvey Young (Knoxville: University of Tennessee Press, 1988), 6–28.

39. William A. Link, *The Paradox of Southern Progressivism, 1880–1930* (Chapel Hill: University of North Carolina Press, 1992), 142–214.

40. T. B. Abercrombie, *History of Public Health in Georgia, 1733–1950* (Atlanta: Georgia Department of Public Health, 1950), 98–99.

41. National Grady Nurses Conclave, box 3. Collins, a 1906 graduate of Spelman, holds the honor of being the only African American nurse whose picture appears in Lavinia Dock's monumental four-volume work, *A History of Nursing* (New York: G. P. Putman's Sons, 1912), 3:176.

42. Abercrombie, *History of Public Health in Georgia,* 107.

43. Louise Tattershall, *Public Health Nursing in the United States, January 15, 1931* (New York: National Organization for Public Health Nurses, 1934), 9, 56.

44. Abercrombie, *History of Public Health in Georgia,* 134–36.

45. Tattershall, *Public Health Nursing*, 18. Of Georgia's 151 public health nurses, 43 were African American.

46. Schissel, "State Nurses' Association," 256.

47. Johns, "A Study," K-14,

48. At least one Georgia patient sympathized with the wish of trained nurses to not work in rural areas. As she reported in Burgess, *Nurses, Patients, and Pocketbooks*, 117, "I live in a country town, and . . . I find that well-equipped and competent nurses, who are accustomed to modern conveniences, [are] unwilling to go into the country in their work. I do not blame them for this, for in the country they have many inconveniences to meet with and usually large crowds of visitors in the patient's room."

49. "Beatrice Parramore," box 3, and "Magnolia Brown," box 1, Georgia Oral History Collection.

50. "Pauline English," box 1, and "Mamie Lee Miller Wilson," box 3, Georgia Oral History Collection.

51. "Laverne Johnson," box 2, Elizabeth Horne," box 2 (also "Betty Kleinstenmber," box 2), and "Alice Latham Herndon," box 1, Georgia Oral History Collection.

52. "Theodora Floyd," box 1, and "Bessie May Dickey," box 1, Georgia Oral History Collection.

53. "Ruth Melber," box 2, and "Lemma Athena Mosely Williamson," box 3, Georgia Oral History Collection. See also "Doris Ada Davis Lovell," box 2, whose sister had gone to training school nine years earlier.

54. "Nillar Orander Almond," box 1; "Birdie Torrance McFarlin," box 2; and "Lena LaVette," box 3, Georgia Oral History Collection.

55. "Rosalie Howell," Atlanta Historical Society, MSS 119.

56. "Nell Hodgson Woodruff Papers, 1913–1982," Manuscript Collection No. 47, Manuscript, Archives, and Rare Book Library, Emory University.

57. President's Report, ANA Southern Division, folder 5, 1933.

58. On Georgia's school system, see Ann Short Chirhart, *Torches of Light: Georgia Teachers and the Coming of the Modern South* (Athens: University of Georgia Press, 2005). Chirhart cites a member of the Rockefeller Foundation's General Education Board who described Georgia in 1925 as "the most primitive state educationally that I have ever been in" (p. 87).

59. See ANA Southern Division, box 1, folder 1, pp. 3–5. These statistics are based on those in Burgess, *Nurses, Patients, and Pocketbooks*, 244.

60. For example, see Johns, "A Study," Exhibit K-15 for the practices of the Atlanta Anti-Tuberculosis Association. As Johns' report makes clear, these practices continued throughout the South.

61. "Lena LaVette," box 2, Georgia Oral History Collection.

62. I am grateful to Carla Schissel's work in this area. See her "State Nurses' Association," 29–51.

63. Data about remaining training schools comes from Rose Broekel Cannon, "Georgia's Twentieth Century Public Health Nurses: A Social History of Racial Relations" (Ph.D. diss., Emory University, 1995). Cannon lists only four: Grady Memorial Hospital (the Municipal Training School); Archibold Memorial Hospital in Thomasville, the University Hospital (Lamar Training School) in Augusta, and the Columbus City Hospital in Columbus. Spelman's training school holds an ambiguous position since its history records that its formal nurses training program (along with its teacher education program) were discontinued in 1928 when Spelman adopted a collegiate focus. Training for African American nurses, however, continued at its affiliated McVicar's Hospital. See www.spelman.edu/about_us/facts/. It is difficult to make national generalizations about where African American women trained as nurses. Many attended schools in African American–run hospitals, but others attended schools in African American hospitals run by white administrators or, as at Grady, in segregated hospitals.

64. Hine, *Black Women in White*.

65. John Dittmer, *Black Georgia in the Progressive Era, 1900–1920* (Urbana: University of Illinois Press, 1977). For an overview of a new approach to the concept of southern progressivism, see Jimmie Franklin's "Blacks and the Progressive Movement: Emergence of a New Synthesis," www.oah.org/pubs/magazine/progressive/franklin.html.

66. Elisabeth Lasch-Quinn, *Black Neighbors: Race and the Limits of Reform in the American Settlement House Movement* (Chapel Hill: University of North Carolina Press), 120–24. For African American churchwomen, see Evelyn Brooks Higginbothum, *Righteous Discontent: The Women's Movement in the Black Baptist Church, 1880–1920* (Cambridge, MA: Harvard University Press, 1993). For Hope's biography, see Jacqueline Anne Rouse, *Lugenia Burns Hope: Black Southern Reformer* (Athens: University of Georgia Press, 1989).

67. Susan L. Smith, *Sick and Tired of Being Sick and Tired: Black Women's Health Activism in America, 1890–1950* (Philadelphia: University of Pennsylvania Press, 1995).

68. See letter of February 24, 1926, of Andrews to Mrs. Kemper Harrold, in Verdelle B. Bellamy, ed., "The History of Grady Memorial Hospital School of Nursing," n.p., National Grady Nurses Conclave, box 7.

69. Grady Hospital Auxiliary Records, May 12, 1931, Georgia State Archives, folder 5.

70. These schools included Freedmen's Hospital in Washington, D.C.; the Lincoln and Harlem Hospitals in New York City; Mercy Hospital in Philadelphia; the Dixie Hospital in Hampton, Virginia; the Hubbard Hospital in Nashville; the Tuskegee Institute in Alabama; and the Provident Hospital in Chicago. Edwin Embree to Ethel Johns, August 13, 1924, Rockefeller Foundation Archives, Record Group 1.1; Series 200; box 121, folder 1504.

71. Johns, "A Study," K-3.

72. Ibid., K-5.

73. Ibid., K-7. Darlene Clark Hine argues that the prevalence of such racist attitudes and deplorable conditions perpetuated a sense of the low status of nursing among educated African Americans, who looked instead to work teaching or in the developing field of social work; see Hine, "The Ethel Johns Report: Black Women in the Nursing Profession," *Journal of Negro History* 67, no. 3 (1982): 212–18.

74. "Lena LaVette," box 2, Georgia Oral History Collection.

75. For an analysis of African American student resistance documented by Johns, see Judith Young, "Revisiting the 1925 Johns Report on African American Nurses," *Nursing History Review* 13 (2005): 91–92.

76. "Birdie Torrance McFarlin," box 2, and "Roberta Roberts Spencer," box 1, Georgia Oral History Collection.

Chapter Six: A Tale of Two Associations: White and African American Nurses in North Carolina

1. Darlene Clark Hine, *Black Women in White: Racial Conflict and Cooperation in the Nursing Profession, 1890–1950* (Bloomington: Indiana University Press, 1989), 184. These principles were recapitulated with reference to their origins in the respective board actions of both the ANA and the NACGN in Hildegarde Peplau's (chair) Report of the American Nurses' Association's Special Committee on Intergroup Relations in May 1960. Copy in Southern Labor Archives, Georgia State University, DCNA Records (hereafter SLA DCNA), box 1777, folder 328.

2. Hine's *Black Women in White*, 162–86, remains the most influential source of this history. See also (Mary) Elizabeth Carnegie, *The Path We Tread: Blacks in Nursing, 1854–1984* (Philadelphia: J. B. Lippincott, 1986).

3. See "NACGN Disbands," in *American Journal of Nursing* 51, no. 3 (1951): 213.

4. Hine, *Black Women in White*, 186.

5. On public health work, see Edward H. Beardsely, *A History of Neglect: Health Care for Blacks and Mill Workers in the 20th Century South* (Knoxville: University of Tennessee Press, 1987): 140–50. On education, see George B. Tin-

dall, *The Emergence of the New South, 1913–1945* (Baton Rouge: Louisiana State University Press, 1967): 495–96.

6. For fuller explanation, see Patricia D'Antonio, "Revisiting and Rethinking the Rewriting of Nursing History," *Bulletin of the History of Medicine* 73 (1999): 268–90.

7. Data on southern nursing leadership has been gathered from Vern L. Bullough, Olga Maranjian Church, and Alice P. Stein, *American Nursing* (New York: Garland Publishing, 1988); Vern L. Bullough, Lilli Sentz, and Alice P. Stein, *American Nursing: A Biographical Dictionary*, Vol. 2 (New York: Garland Publishing, 1992); and Adah Thoms's early history, *Pathfinders: A History of the Progress of Colored Graduate Nurses, with Biographies of Many Prominent Nurses* (New York: Kay Printing House, 1929). Of the nurses whose birthplaces were noted, 50 percent (11/22) were born in the South, but only 9 percent (2/22) were trained in southern nursing schools. As with white nurses, where one trained seems more important than class background, since most of prominent early twentieth-century African American nurses were trained at Provident Hospital in Chicago, Lincoln Hospital in New York City, Freedmen's Hospital in Washington, D.C., Mercy Hospital in Philadelphia, or the Kansas City General Hospital #2. Only 17 percent trained in southern hospitals, most notably Dixie Hospital in Hampton, Virginia, and the Tuskegee Institute in Alabama.

8. Ellen D. Baer, "American Nursing: 100 Years of Conflicting Ideas and Ideals, *Journal of the New York State Nurses' Association* 23, no. 3 (1992): 16–21.

9. See "Memorandum" dated August 20, 1938, in SLA DCNA, box 1777/328, "historical files."

10. Josephine Pitman Prescott to Asby Taylor, April 23, 1947, SLA DCNA, box 1777/328, "historical files."

11. Asby Taylor to Josephine Pitman Prescott, April 27, 1947, SLA DCNA, box 1777/328, "historical files."

12. See, for example, Mabel Staupers to Miss Beattie (GNA), April 27, 1945, and Mabel Staupers to Miss McIver (ANA), January 30, 1945, SLA DCNA, box 1777/328, "historical files."

13. See, for example, Agnes Dean (ANA) to Gertrude Bowling (GNA), March 30, 1926, SLA DCNA, box 1777/328, "historical files."

14. North Carolina State Nurses Association (NCSNA), North Carolina State Archives, 1929.

15. For example, among Thoms's prominent nurses in *Pathfinders*, only 26 percent ultimately chose careers in southern states. For data on southern nurses not wanting to return, see Marjorie Stimson and Louise Tattershall, "A Study of Negro Public Health Nursing," *Public Health Nurse*, October 1930, 531–32.

16. Mary Lewis Wyche, *The History of Nursing in North Carolina* (Chapel Hill: University of North Carolina, 1938), 109.

17. See data from the Raleigh Women's Club, 1924, when reporting on their visit to the Rex Hospital, North Carolina State Archives.

18. North Carolina State Nurses Association (NCSNA), North Carolina State Archives, 1926.

19. The official mantra endorsed by white nurses representing not only North Carolina but all the southern states in the ANA was that the "the nursing profession will never rise any higher than the status of whatever group it neglects." See Alma Haupt, Discussion of Mrs. Riddle's Paper, ANA Southern Division, 1935.

20. NCSNA, 1919.

21. "Rubye Bowles Bryson," quoted in Jane Abernathy Plyler, "Public Health Nursing in North Carolina: Oral Histories of Earlier Years" (master's thesis, University of North Carolina, Chapel Hill School of Public Health, 1980), 36.

22. See "Shirley Titus," in *Dictionary of American Nursing Biography* (New York: Greenwood Press, 1988): 369–70.

23. Shirley Titus, "Present Trends in Nursing Education," ANA Southern Division, 1935, 39–47. Quotes on 44, 42, and 47, respectively.

24. See, for example, Lavinia Dock, "Status of the Nurse in the Working World," *American Journal of Nursing* 13 (1913): 971.

25. See, for example, Alma Eldridge, "The Need for a Sound Professional Preparation for Colored Nurses," *Proceedings of the Annual Congress on Medical Education, Medical Licensure, and Hospitals* 94, no. 18 (1930): 168–71.

26. ANA Southern Division, 1935. The capitalization was in Riddle's prepared presentation in SD records.

27. Ibid.

28. Ibid. James Weldon Johnson is perhaps best known as the co-composer, with his brother, of "Lift Every Voice and Sing," quickly adopted as the Negro National Anthem.

29. State Association of Negro Registered Nurses (SANRN), North Carolina State Archives, 1923–1925.

30. Ibid., 1933.

31. For more information on these projects, see Jeffrey J. Crow, Paul D. Escott, and Flora J. Holley, *History of African Americans in North Carolina* (Raleigh: North Carolina Department of Resources, Division of Archives and History, 1992), 136–37.

32. For African American club women in North Carolina, see Glenda Elizabeth Gilmore's *Gender and Jim Crow: Women and the Politics of White Supremacy in*

North Carolina, 1896-1920 (Chapel Hill: University of North Carolina Press, 1996).

33. For African American health activism in the South, see Susan L. Smith, *Sick and Tired of Being Sick and Tired: Black Women's Health Activism in America, 1890-1950* (Philadelphia: University of Pennsylvania Press, 1995).

34. Ruth Anita Hawkins Hughes, *Contributions of Vance County People of Color* (Henderson, NC: Sparks Press, 1988), 401.

35. SANRN, 1930.

36. Ibid., 1923.

37. The 1931 National Organization for Public Health Nursing (NOPHN) survey of public health nurses cited only 20 African American public health nurses practicing in North Carolina and only 211 practicing in the states that made up the Southern Division. See Louise Tattershall, *Public Health Nursing in the United States, 1931* (New York: National Organization for Public Health Nursing, 1934). For salary differentials, see SANRN, 1941. White public health nurses were paid between $100 and $110, while African American salaries were $75 to $90.

38. "Edith MacNeil Holmes," in Plyler, "Public Health Nursing in North Carolina," 53.

39. Thompson makes specific reference to the infighting done when visitors were present. The proceedings indicate these visitors are representatives from the State Board of Health (SANRN, 1937).

40. NCSNA, 1940.

41. SANRN, 1943.

42. NCSNA, 1944. This letter is not mentioned in the SANRN minutes, and the minutes for 1944 are missing.

43. NCSNA, 1946. On Florida, see Carnegie's *The Path We Tread*, 90.

44. See Beardsely, *History of Neglect*, 177–84, for a discussion of Hill-Burton planning in the South in general, and North Carolina in particular.

45. NCSNA, 1946.

46. Ibid., 1948.

47. Ibid., 1946.

48. For example, see Mary Duke Biddle Trent Seman's role as a trustee of the African American Lincoln Hospital and a member of the Hill-Burton's Committee of One Hundred that worked to ensure equitable distribution of monies to African American hospitals, in "Semans Family Papers, Mary Duke Biddle Trent Seman," Duke University Special Collections, finding aid, 25.

49. NCSAN, 1947; SANRN, 1947.

50. NCSNA Board of Directors Meeting, October 1948, North Carolina State Archives, 1948.

51. There is a vibrant scholarship on African American women and their construction of gender in the context of race and racism and about their linking their commitment to individual achievement with that of their community. For a review, see Linda Alexander's "The Challenge of Race: Rethinking the Position of Black Women in the Field of Women's History," *Journal of Women's History* 16 (2004): 50–60. For a more direct consideration of black women professionals, see Stephanie Shaw, *What a Woman Ought to Be and Do: Black Professional Women Workers During the Jim Crow Era* (Chicago: University of Chicago Press, 1996).

52. "Elizabeth McMillan Thompson," in Plyler, "Public Health Nursing in North Carolina," 100.

53. This cost-cutting was across the board in terms of state budget in the 1930s, but given salary differentials, it hit African American nurses hardest.

54. "Elizabeth McMillan Thompson," in Plyler, "Public Health Nursing in North Carolina," 101.

55. Mary Elizabeth Carnegie, "The Path We Tread," *International Nursing Review* 9 (September-October 1962): 25–33.

56. NCSNA, 1948, 47.

57. Ibid., 42–43.

58. Ibid., 42.

59. Ibid., 42.

60. Ibid., 47.

61. SANRN, June 1948.

62. Ibid., November 1948.

63. Ibid., 1949.

64. "Edith MacNeil Holmes," in Plyler, "Public Health Nursing in North Carolina," 53.

65. Rhonda L. Goldstein, "Negro Nurses in Hospitals," *American Journal of Nursing* 60, no. 2 (1960): 216.

66. This was not a uniquely southern phenomenon. Alma Scott, the ANA representative to the Southern Division in 1943, spoke of organizational resentment of nurses aide programs throughout the country set up "by a bunch of rich society women who want their names in the newspapers." See ANA Southern Division, 1943.

67. See Beardsely, *History of Neglect*, 251–53. In 1954 the North Carolina Medical Association offered "scientific membership" to the African American physicians of the Old North State Medical Society. The Old North State Medical

Society rejected the offer and censured the two black physicians who took advantage of it. Segregation continued in North Carolina medical organizations through the early 1960s. By contrast, African American physicians did accept the Memphis and Shelby County Medical Society's offer of "scientific membership" only in 1955. See Keith Wailoo, *Dying in the City of the Blues: Sickle Cell Anemia and the Politics of Race* (Chapel Hill: University of North Carolina Press, 2000), 114.

68. Marie B. Noell, "If You Ask Me . . . ," *American Journal of Nursing* 63, no. 9 (1963): 64.

69. Mary Elizabeth Carnegie and Estelle Massey Riddle, "Integration in Professional Nursing," *Crisis* 69 (January 1962): 5–9.

70. "Edith MacNeil Holmes," in Plyler, "Public Health Nursing in North Carolina," 56.

Chapter Seven: Who Is a Nurse?

1. William D. White, ed., introduction to *Compelled by Data: John Devereaux Thompson, Nurse, Health Services Researcher, and Health Administration Educator,* http://info.med.yale.edu/eph/pdf/Thompson.pdf (retrieved 8 December 2008). Thompson was also a noted historian. He and colleague Grace Goldin had published the landmark book, *The Hospital: A Social and Architectural History* (New Haven, CT: Yale University Press, 1975).

2. Donna Diers, personal communication, July 16, 2009.

3. Edward J. Halloran, "John Devereaux Thompson, RN, MS," in *Compelled by Data*, 23.

4. Ibid., 2.

5. Allen Ernst to Leroy Craig, December 15, 1925, Archives of the Pennsylvania Hospital Training School for Men, box 2, folder 2, The Pennsylvania Hospital, Philadelphia. Craig was the superintendent of its men's training school.

6. See, for example, Frederick Jones's "Opportunity for Men Nurses," and Frances Witte's survey in "Opportunities in Graduate Education for Men Nurses," in *American Journal of Nursing*, 34, no. 4 (1934): 131–33.

7. National Center for Educational Statistics, *120 Years of Education: A Statistical Profile,* U.S. Department of Education, Office of Educational Research and Improvement, January 1993, Table 2: School Enrollment of 5–19-year-olds per 100 persons, by sex and race: 1850 to 1991, p. 14. Available online at http://nces.ed.gov/pubs93/93442.pdf.

8. Historical Abstracts of the United States, No. HS-30 Marital Status of Women in the Civilian Labor Force: 1900–2002. Available online at www.census.gov/statab/hist/HS-30pdf (retrieved 10 July 2008).

9. Ibid.

10. www.census.gov/population/socdemo/education/tableA-2.txt (retrieved 6 August 2008).

11. Susan Reverby, *Ordered to Care: The Dilemma of American Nursing, 1850–1945* (New York: Cambridge University Press, 1987), 177; Darlene Clark Hine, *Black Women in White: Racial Conflict and Cooperation in the Nursing Profession, 1890–1950* (Bloomington: Indiana University Press, 1989), 108.

12. Frances Helen Zeigler, "Relief Unemployment," *American Journal of Nursing* 34, no. 8 (1934): 761.

13. Jean C. Whelan, "'A Necessity in the Nursing World': The Chicago Nurses Professional Registry, 1913–1950," *Nursing History Review* 13 (2004): 58–62.

14. Philip A. Kalisch and Beatrice J. Kalisch, *The Advance of American Nursing*, 3rd ed. (Philadelphia: J. B. Lippincott, 1995), 312.

15. Hine, *Black Women in White*, 124.

16. For information on the *Farmer's Wife*, see www.time.com/time/magazine/article/0,9171,758987,00.html.

17. "About the Boltons," in Robert Lewis Bolton Papers, #4043, box 5, folder #33, Southern Historical Collection, Library of the University of North Carolina at Chapel Hill.

18. "Reminiscences of Florence Jacob Edmunds," Butler Library, Columbia University, Black Women Oral History Project, NXCP87-A669.

19. Edmunds went on to a prominent career in nursing and, after her retirement, to community volunteer work establishing community day care for African American children, serving as the first African American board member of the local Salvation Army chapter and of the local museum. Her contributions were honored with her selection as Pittsfield's "Mother of the Year" in 1962 and as the focus of a "This is Your Life" tribute in 1975.

20. For information on the Cadet Nurse Corps, see http://lhncbc.nlm.nih.gov/apdb/phsHistory/resources/cadetnurse/nurse05.html. See also Thelma Robinson and Paulien M. Perry, *Cadet Nurse Stories: The Call for and Response of Women During World War II* (Indianapolis, IN: Center Nursing Publishing, 2001).

21. Julie Fairman and Joan Lynaugh, *Critical Care Nursing: A History* (Philadelphia: University of Pennsylvania Press, 1998); Arlene Keeling, "Blurring the Boundaries Between Medicine and Nursing: Cardiac Care Nursing, Circa the 1960s," *Nursing History Review* 13 (2005): 139–64.

22. Kalish and Kalish, *Advance of American Nursing*, 504.

23. Ibid., 370.

24. Ibid., 378–79.

25. Esther Lucile Brown, *Nursing for the Future: A Report Prepared for the National Nursing Council* (New York: Russell Sage Foundation, 1948), 27–33.

26. Joan Lynaugh, "Nursing the Great Society: The Impact of the Nurse Training Act of 1964," *Nursing History Review* 16 (2008): 13–28.

27. Kalish and Kalish, *Advance of American Nursing*, 448.

28. See Patricia T. Haase, *The Origins and Rise of Associate Degree Nursing Education* (Durham, NC: National League for Nursing and Duke University Press, 1990).

29. Catherine Cenzia Choy, *Empire of Care: Nursing and Migration in Filipino American History* (Durham, NC: Duke University Press, 2003), esp. 10–12.

30. Eileen Sullivan Marx, "A Conversation with Louise Smith, RN: The First Hopi Trained Nurse," Barbara Bates Center for the Study of the History of Nursing. See also the life and nursing career of Edith Leroy Richardson, the granddaughter of a Uintah Utes chief, in Edith Leroy Richardson Papers, 1883–1971, University of Utah Special Collections, MS 366. For a contemporary's perspective on the relationship between white trained nurses and American Indians, see Elinor Gregg, *The Indian and the Nurse* (Norman: University of Oklahoma Press, 1965). See also Mary Ann Ruffing-Rahal, "The Navajo Experience of Elizabeth Forster, Public Health Nurse," *Nursing History Review* 3 (1995): 173–89.

31. Annie Soo, "The Life and Career of Minnie Lee Fong," in Jack Chen, *The Chinese of America* (San Francisco: Harper & Row, 1987), 67–71. Judy Yung also briefly discusses the careers of Alice Fong Yu and Minnie Fong Lee in *Unbound Feet: A Social History of Chinese Women in San Francisco* (Berkeley: University of California Press, 1995), 141–42.

32. Thomas Dublin, *Transforming Women's Work: New England Lives in the Industrial Revolution* (Ithaca, NY: Cornell University Press, 1994).

33. National Center for Education Statistics, "Digest of Education Statistics: 2007," available at http://nces.ed.gov/programs/digest/d07/tables/dt07_008 .asp?referrer=list (retrieved 18 December 2008).

34. Luther Chrisman, "Who Is a nurse?" *Image: The Journal of Nursing Scholarship* 30, no. 3 (1998): 211–14 (quote on page 211).

35. Jerome Lysaught, *From Abstract to Action: National Committee for the Study of Nursing and Nursing Education* (New York: McGraw Hill, 1973), 140–41.

36. *The Registered Nurse Population: Findings from the March 2004 National Sample Survey of Registered Nurses*, Table 40, U.S. Department of Health and Human Services, Health Resources and Services Administration,

available at http://bhpr.hrsa.gov/healthworkforce/rnsurvey04/ (retrieved 10 October 2007).

37. Ibid., Table 33.

38. See statistics of the Women Physicians Congress at www.ama-assn.org/ama/pub/category/12912.html.

As I THINK ABOUT THE scholarship that has informed my approach to the history of nursing, I feel something like an archeologist systematically surveying the texts in my bookcases, excavating hidden gems that I have not thought about in quite some time, and articulating connections between the exemplary work of those who have come before me and my own interpretations. This essay is by no means exhaustive. Researchers writing about nursing's history from positions both within and outside of the discipline have produced a rich body of studies about individuals, training schools and colleges, animating ideas, and actual practices. A survey of the articles published in the volumes of the *Nursing History Review,* the official journal of the American Association for the History of Nursing, and in *Nursing Inquiry* provides immediate access to the breadth and depth of this particular field of inquiry. Both journals provide a space where scholars from many different disciplines come together to explore the ways in which the histories of nurses and nursing intersect with histories that explore the possibilities and the problems of fundamental human importance around the globe.

This essay, by contrast, allows me to acknowledge my personal intellectual debts. Like any good archeologist, then, I must return to the beginning: to M. Adelaide Nutting and Lavinia L. Dock's magisterial four-volume *A History of Nursing* (New York: G. P. Putnam's Sons, 1907–1912). Nutting and Dock's explicit intent was to make visible what had been invisible. And their rationale still echoes in many histories of nursing today. They wanted to counter "long ages of silence" about gentler and more humane acts that made human society possible, to challenge "the tendency of historians to overlook what was usual and homely," and to show nurses how their history was inexorably linked with that of other women. "As they rise," they wrote, "she rises, and as they sink, she falls."

The first two volumes, both published in 1907, take the reader on a stirring sweep of *The Evolution of Nursing Systems from the Earliest Times to the Foundation of the First English and American Training Schools for Nurses.* We travel from the caregiving of preliterate peoples to that of ancient Greece and Rome. We track the care available in families to that available in the rising religious orders. We dread the eighteenth century's "dark period," which coincided with the general subjugation of women. Yet we revel in the nineteenth century's revival, presaged by the German deaconate and fulfilled in the triumphs of Florence Nightingale. Dock edited the last two volumes, *From Earliest Times to the Present Day with Special Reference to the Work of the Past Thirty Years.* Both were published in 1912, and both contained essays by nurses around the globe describing the emergence of trained nursing in their respective countries. These volumes take their readers on tours of nursing in Japan and China, into leper colonies in the Philippines, and into the Cama Hospital in Bombay. Most of the stories are of white nursing women sponsored by religious missions and colonial governments and charged with the care of indigenous peoples. But the reader sees hope for the future in proud pictures of small graduating classes of native-born women in such places as Syria, Korea, and Cuba.

There is much that we, with more modern eyes, might point to as wrong about Dock and Nutting's *A History of Nursing.* It is about great women doing great things within the great sweep of historical time. Dock and Nutting and their various contributors are themselves blind to their privileges of race and class. Their enshrinement of the "trio of training schools"—those at the Bellevue Hospital in New York City, at the New Haven Hospital in Connecticut, and at the Massachusetts General Hospital in Boston—as those from which the steady march of nursing progress in America dates has long obscured the important role played by earlier nurses training initiatives.

Yet one cannot help but be moved by Dock and Nutting's passion, optimism, confidence, and intellect. They were the true children of their era: progressives certain that the rational application of knowledge would lead to substantive change; educated women asserting their right to power and a public voice; and clinicians, like their medical colleagues at Johns Hopkins, seeking to harness their history in service to their newly articulated claims to scientific authority. Diane Hamilton, in "Constructing the Mind of Nursing" (*Nursing History Review* 2 [1994]: 3–28), places these women in an early twentieth-century "thought collective" that intellectually reified compassion as one of the basic guiding principles of the new discipline. But for me, their powerful narrative demanded that I take them, their ideas, their institutions, and their vision seriously. It also shaped how I came to look for and understand the ways in which nurses created and maintained a powerful and shared internal identity that served as a defense against social perceptions that often belied their sense of themselves. Not surprisingly, *A History of Nursing* was condensed into a one-volume text in 1920. The renamed *A Short History of Nursing* (New York: G. P. Putnam's Sons, 1920) quickly became required reading for generations of nursing students.

By mid-century, the pride of place held by *A History of Nursing* yielded to other authors and other perspectives. Some, like Victor Robinson in *White Caps: The Story of Nursing* (1946) and Richard Shyrock in *History of Nursing, an Interpretation of the Social and Medical Factors Involved* (1959) were constructed by physicians turning to the history of nursing after completing works on the history of medicine. Most, however, were written by nurses looking toward nurses as their primary audience. Mary Roberts, then editor of the *American Journal of Nursing*, published *American Nursing: History and Interpretation* (1954), which, not surprisingly, focused on the place of leaders and leading institutions in the history of nursing. Josephine Dolan's varyingly titled histories of nursing held prominence from the 1960s through the 1980s.[3] These texts favored facts over interpretative leaps. But historians who tend toward more analytic work can often overlook the critical importance of factually accurate texts. The varying editions of texts by Philip A. Kalish and Beatrice J. Kalish have been particularly useful in my own work. I have depended heavily on the third edition of *The Advance of American Nursing* (Philadelphia: J. B. Lippincott, 1986).

But at the same time that these texts were rolling off publishers' presses, the field of nursing history was in the process of a profound transformation. If the triumphant *A History of Nursing* was the first book I read, Jo Ann Ashley's devastating *Hospitals, Paternalism and the Role of the Nurse* (New York: Teachers College Press, 1976) was the second. Ashley unfurled a furious—and controversial—critique of the sexism of male physicians and hospital administrators that had kept nurses subservient for generations. Like *A History of Nursing*, it was a work of passion. But unlike its early twentieth-century predecessor, Ashley's historical nurses were curiously passive and even complicit in their own subordination.

This theme of subordination runs through some of the more recent studies on the history of nursing. Mary Poovey's classic argument in *Uneven Developments: The Ideological Work of Gender in Mid-Victorian England* (University of Chicago Press, 1988) that nursing never realized its potentially subversive threat to gendered roles still carries weight. The Nightingale-inspired positioning of women nurses in a traditionally hierarchical ordering vis-à-vis male physicians, she argued, signaled an end to a battle over roles before it had even

---

[3] Dolan began collaborating with Minnie Goodnow on her *History of Nursing* in 1958. She began editing what then became *Goodnow's History of Nursing* in 1960. Dolan subsequently published *Nursing in Society: A Historical Perspective* in 1968 and took it through thirteen editions until she herself turned to M. Louise Fitzpatrick and Eleanor Kron Herrmann as collaborators in 1983. W. B. Saunders of Philadelphia published all these editions.

begun. Joan Roberts and Thetis Group's *Feminism and Nursing: An Historical Perspective on Power, Status, and Political Activism in the Nursing Profession* (Westport, CT: Praeger, 1995) and their later *Nursing, Physician Control, and the Medical Monopoly* (Bloomington: Indiana University Press, 2001) return to this theme, but unfortunately with more of Ashley's stridency than Poovey's nuances. A more insightful iteration of the theme of subordination can be seen in the work of literary theorist Kristine Swenson, who borrows Poovey's methodological combination of historical and textural analysis. In *Medical Women and Victorian Fiction* (Columbia: University of Missouri Press, 2005), Swenson's "New Woman" doctors emerge as more significant actors than nurses in shaping Britain's late nineteenth-century medical practice because they more easily rejected the ideology of separate spheres of influence in the process of becoming emancipated professionals.

Florence Nightingale, of course, remains the lightening rod in these analyses. Few actors have captured historians' attention to the extent that she has. There seems to be a biography that matches one's mood. If you feel quietly congratulatory, read Cecil Woodham-Smith's well-regarded *Florence Nightingale, 1820–1910* (London: Constable Press, 1950). If you feel rather cross about her influence, turn to F. B. Smith's manipulative and self-aggrandizing villain in *Florence Nightingale: Reputation and Power* (London: Croom Helm, 1982). And if you feel rather pressed for time, pick up the remarkable yet underrated collection of essays in Vern Bullough, Bonnie Bullough, and Marietta Stanton's *Florence Nightingale and Her Era: A Collection of New Scholarship* (New York: Garland Publishing, 1990).

More recently, researchers have tended to focus on particular moments in Nightingale's life. Hugh Small, in *Florence Nightingale: Avenging Angel* (New York: St. Martin's Press, 1999) focuses on her time in the Crimea and her deep distress when she discovered that the mortality rates at her own hospital in Scutari were higher than those at British hospitals elsewhere in the region. Monica Baly's *Florence Nightingale and the Nursing Legacy* (London: Whurr, 1997) turns to the famous nurses' training school at St. Thomas' in London and suggests that much of its success came from a well-oiled publicity machine. Jharna Gourlay's *Florence Nightingale and the Health of the Raj* (Farnham, UK: Ashgate, 2003) focuses on Nightingale's involvement with India and charts her movement from a narrow focus only on the health of the British Army to a much broader perspective that supported political changes as a means to address the subcontinent's social and economic concerns. Gillian Gill's *Nightingales: The Extraordinary Upbringing and Curious Life of Miss Florence Nightingale* (New York: Ballantine, 2004) returns to Nightingale's childhood and suggest that far from being an enigma to a staunchly bourgeois family, Nightingale grew up surrounded by a warm circle of intellectually curious, socially committed, and strong women.

We have long needed a new full-length biography of Nightingale. It has been more than thirty years since anyone has risen to the challenge of sifting through newly found letters and stale historiographic debates. And a fabulous one has just appeared in Mark Bostridge's *Florence Nightingale: The Making of an Icon* (New York: Farrar, Straus and Giroux, 2008). Bostridge's Nightingale is neither a heroine nor a harpy. She is a fully formed character who perhaps loved the abstraction of humanity more than the idiosyncrasies of individual humans. Bostridge advances no new thesis or argument about the meaning of Nightingale's life and stunning achievements. Rather, he creates a compelling story of a complicated woman who might well be aghast at how she has come to represent so many different things to so many different people.

Of course, one need not take a particular author's word on any aspect of Nightingale's life. A rich body of work allows Nightingale to speak for herself, using her own books and letters to directly engage a reader. Her *Notes on Nursing, Notes on Hospitals*, and *Cassandra* have long been available both as valuable first editions and as more accessible reprints. But her *Suggestions for Thought*, a massive opus privately printed in 1860, never found an audience. The book, her friends told her, needed editing. But it did not find its editors until 1994, when Michael Calabria and Janet Macrae published their *Suggestions for Thought by Florence Nightingale: Selections and Commentaries* (Philadelphia: University of Pennsylvania Press). It is one thing to read that Nightingale was well-educated, religiously minded, and firmly convinced of the righteousness of her cause. It is quite another to actually experience it and to fully realize the scope of her intellect and the depth of her convictions. I have also particularly enjoyed Martha Vicinus and Bea Nergaard's *Ever Yours, Florence Nightingale: Selected Letters* (1990) and Sue Goldie's *Florence Nightingale: Letters from the Crimea* (Cambridge: Harvard University Press, 1997) for the way they document the development of a woman discovering not only how much she loved the taste of official power but also how much good she could do with it. Lynn McDonald's project to publish all of Nightingale's surviving personal letters, professional reports, formal books, and scribbled notes is both more ambitious—and more contentious—than these other collections. Eleven of a projected sixteen volumes have been published. McDonald and her collaborators have organized Nightingale's writings thematically rather than chronologically. These volumes allow a reader to trace Nightingale's evolving ideas around such themes as spirituality, the role of women, public health, and Indian reform. But they assume discrete boundaries around particular concerns that may or may not have been apparent to Nightingale, and one does lose a sense of how these selected themes intersected with each other and with the sometimes ordinariness of a life that even Nightingale led.[4]

I had once thought that I too might join the pantheon of Nightingale scholars. Fortunately, wise counsel steered me to the then new and exciting work of social historians mining the history of nursing for what it might suggest about the intersections of gender, class, race, work, and the meaning of professionalism in women's lives. Through the 1980s, five scholars, working contemporaneously, defined the field in the United States. Janet Wilson James's "Isabel Hampton and the Professionalization of Nursing in the 1890s" (1979) took a more nuanced look at one of the most important leaders of the American nursing's professionalizing project.[5] Barbara Melosh, by contrast, in *"The Physician's Hand": Work Culture and Conflict in American Nursing* (Philadelphia: Temple University Press, 1982) turned her attention to the heretofore invisible work culture of the vast majority of "ordinary" or "rank and file" nurses and highlighted the power of nurses' craft traditions as they negotiated the often troubled terrain of paid labor. Susan Armeny's dissertation, "Resolute Enthusiasts: The Effort to Professionalize American Nursing, 1880–1915" (Columbia: University of Missouri, 1983), contrasted these women and their concerns about economic security in their day-to-day working lives with the professionalizing ambitions of their ostensible leaders, women like Nutting and Dock, who chose nursing as a way to bring meaning, power, autonomy, and status into their lives. This juxtaposition of craft traditions with professionalizing rhetoric continues to inform some histories of nursing, most recently Tom Olson and Eileen Walsh's *Handling the Sick: The Women of St. Luke's and the Nature of Nursing, 1892–1937* (Columbus: Ohio State University Press, 2004). But Jean Whelan's dissertation, "Too Many, Too Few: The Supply, Demand, and Distribution of Private Duty Nurses, 1910–1965" (University of Pennsylvania, 2000) breaks down such divisions and suggests more leadership support for rank and file agendas than has been previously acknowledged.

My own work has been more directly framed by Susan Reverby's enormously influential *Ordered to Care: The Dilemma of American Nursing, 1850–1945* (New York: Cambridge University Press, 1987). Reverby also positioned nurses as workers. But she framed caring as the most important form of that work and then placed that work within the broader history of the political economy of the evolving American hospital. Her story was one of constraints: of women ordered

---

[4]A description of the project and the volumes available through Wilfrid Laurier University Press is available at www.sociology.uoguelph.ca/fnightingale.

[5]In Ellen D. Boer, Patricia D'Antonio, Sylvia Rinker, and Joan Lynaugh, eds., *Enduring Issues in American Nursing* (New York: Springer, 2001).

to care in a society that refused to value caring, and of women caught in the socially constructed bind of perceiving altruism as the antithesis of autonomy and trapped there by class divisions that precluded the development of any new ideology based on gender. Reverby's hard-hitting analysis foregrounded gender and class. Darlene Clark Hine, by contrast, did so with gender and race. Her *Black Women in White: Racial Conflict and Cooperation in the Nursing Profession, 1890-1950* (Bloomington: Indiana University Press, 1989) built on such works as Adah Thoms's *Pathfinders: A History of the Progress of Colored Graduate Nurses* (New York: Kay Printing House, 1929), Mabel Staupers's *No Time for Prejudice: A Story of the Integration of Negroes in Nursing in the United States* (New York: Macmillan, 1961) and M. Elizabeth Carnegie's *The Path We Tread: Blacks in Nursing Worldwide, 1854-1994* (Philadelphia: Lippincott, 1986). These authors also figure as important actors in my history. But Hine's study was more conceptual and argued that even as African American nurses contended with their own divisive class issues, they remained joined both by choice and by institutional and social racism to a community beyond that of their hospitals.

Scholars either located across the globe or interested in issues beyond the borders of the United States also experimented with the implications of this "new nursing history." Brian Able-Smith's *A History of the Nursing Profession* (London: Heinemann, 1975), Christopher Maggs's *The Origins of General Nursing* (London: Croom Helm, 1983), Judith Moore's *A Zeal for Responsibility: The Struggle for Professional Nursing in Victorian England, 1868-1883* (Athens: University of Georgia Press, 1988), and Anne Marie Rafferty's *The Politics of Nursing Knowledge* (London: Routledge, 1996) brought this perspective to different themes in the history of nursing in the United Kingdom. Katherine McPherson's *Bedside Matters: The Transformation of Canadian Nursing, 1900-1990* (Toronto: Oxford University Press, 1996) created Canada's first social history of nursing, and Gerard Fealy's *A History of Apprenticeship Nurse Training in Ireland: Bright Faces and Neat Dresses* (London: Routledge, 2005) did so for Ireland. Joan Lynaugh and Barbara Brush's *Nurses of All Nations: A History of the International Council of Nurses, 1899-1999* (Philadelphia: Williams and Wilkins, 1999) focused attention on one of the earliest women's international associations.

The role of the state is one emerging theme in these particular histories that begs further analysis. Historians who have studied international communities of nurses with more centralized national governments have long argued that interest in and support for nursing's reform initiatives have often been for reasons that have little to do with only ensuring improvements in health care services. For example, Shula Marks's *Divided Sisterhood: Race, Class and Gender in the South African Nursing Profession* (London: Palgrave Macmillan, 1994) suggests that the South African state championed the professionalizing aspirations of nursing as a remarkably effective tool to create a stable, bourgeois middle class that might support the policies of the apartheid government. Likewise, Katrin Schultheiss's *Bodies and Souls: Politics and the Professionalization of Nursing in France, 1880–1922* (Cambridge: Harvard University Press, 2001) argues that the government of the Third Republic promoted reforms in nursing education and practice as part of a policy to diminish the influence of the Roman Catholic Church in general, and the religious nursing sisterhoods in particular. Catherine Cenzia Choy's *Empire of Care: Nursing and Migration in Filipino American History* (Durham: Duke University Press, 2003) places nurses at the nexus of one country's export economy and another's import one. And Bronwyn Rebekah McFarland-Icke's *Nurses in Nazi Germany: Moral Choice in History* (Princeton University Press, 1999) turns caring on its head with nurses as actors in their country's T4 program to extinguish lives not worth living.

But as studies of nursing in the military show, nurses were never passive victims of state interests. Anne Summers' *Angels and Citizens: British Women as Military Nurses, 1854–1914* (London: Routledge and Kegan Paul, 1988) established a new interpretive paradigm in which military nursing corps became the only place where women could participate in the great events of their time in positions of responsibility and personal challenge. This place was not without its own contradictions. Cynthia Toman's *An Officer and a Lady: Canadian Military Nursing and the Second World War* (Vancouver: University of British Columbia Press, 2007) continues to develop the tensions that existed between commitments to healing within the slaughter of war. Jane Schultz's *Women at the Front: Hospital Workers in Civil War America* (Chapel Hill: University of North Carolina Press, 2004) aptly captures the ways groups of women replicated the same race and class hierarchies within the military that they had known in their own communities at home. Mary Sarnecky's encyclopedic *A History of the U.S. Army Nurse Corps* (Philadelphia: University of Pennsylvania Press, 1999) provides entry into the breadth of what were exclusively women's experiences until 1954, when men were also allowed to serve as army nurses. Elizabeth Norman's *We Band of Angels: The Untold Story of American Nurses Trapped on Bataan by the Japanese* (New York: Random House, 1999) and Evelyn Monahan and Rosemary Neidel-Greenlee's *And If I Perish: Frontline U.S. Army Nurses in World War II* (New York: Knopf, 2003) speak of these women's enduring hold on the public imagination.

The past decade has seen a shift away from interpretive sweeps of time, places, and events to more nuanced analyses of nursing practice. These works seriously engage the constraint and contradiction theses that have dominated the recent historiography. Yet they also suggest that such were neither nonnegotiable nor insurmountable. Julie Fairman and Joan Lynaugh's *Critical Care Nursing: A History* (Philadelphia: University of Pennsylvania, 1998), and Julie Fairman's *Making Room in the Clinic: Nurse Practitioners and the Evolution of Modern Health Care* (New Brunswick, NJ: Rutgers University Press, 2008) show how grass-roots alliances with supportive physicians and other health care reformers allowed ambitious nurses to successfully push the boundaries of clinical practice in hospital-based intensive care units and in community-based primary care settings. Margarete Sandelowski's *Devices and Desires: Gender, Technology, and American Nursing* (Chapel Hill: University of North Carolina Press, 2000) and Arlene Keeling's *Nursing and the Privilege of Prescription, 1893–2000* (Columbus: Ohio State University Press, 2007) similarly argue that nurses quietly assumed the right to particular practices that physicians believed to be their prerogatives.

Other scholars have turned their attention to areas of nursing work that had long been invisible, and position the practices of their nurses as absolutely central to the larger histories of institutions and of health care practices and policy. Sioban Nelson's *Say Little, Do Much: Nurses, Nuns, and Hospitals in the Nineteenth Century* (Philadelphia: University of Pennsylvania Press, 2001) and Barbra Mann Wall's *Unlikely Entrepreneurs: Catholic Sisters and the Hospital Marketplace, 1865–1925* (Columbus: Ohio State University Press, 2005) turn to the work of vowed women nurses and gives us a more nuanced and gendered story of hospital formation. Joan Lynaugh and Barbara Brush's *American Nursing: From Hospitals to Health Care Systems* (Hoboken, NJ: Wiley-Blackwell, 1997) places nurses at the center of the later twentieth-century health system movement. Cynthia Connolly, in *Saving Sickly Children: The Tuberculosis Preventorium in American Life, 1909–1970* (New Brunswick, NJ: Rutgers University Press, 2008), places nurses at the nexus of struggles to develop family welfare policies and public health practices for children considered "at risk" of the White Plague of tuberculosis. Karen Buhler-Wilkerson's *False Dawn: The Rise and Decline of Public Health Nursing, 1900–1930* (New York: Garland, 1990) and her later *No Place Like Home: A History of Nursing and Home Care in the United States* (Baltimore: Johns Hopkins University Press, 2001) draw on the experiences of nurses to examine how the complicated intersections of race, ethnicity, types of illnesses, and particularities of place influenced who had access to what kinds of care in their own homes. Buhler-Wilkerson's emphasis on place has been particularly influential in my own work.

Biographies have been another important genre. As Laurel Thatcher Ulrich and Emily K. Abel have so brilliantly shown in their respective *A Midwife's Tale: The Life of Martha Ballard, Based on Her Diary, 1785–1812* (New York: Knopf, 1990) and *Hearts of Wisdom: American Women Caring for Kin, 1850–1940*

(Cambridge: Harvard University Press, 2000), we now have a richer awareness of the many ways in which women lived their lives enmeshed in the simultaneity of their roles as midwives, nurses, mothers, spouses, neighbors, and friends. We also have a deeper understanding of the ways in which nursing played a very prominent role in the lives of women who are remembered for different kinds of legacies. Elizabeth Pryor's *Clara Barton: Professional Angel* (Philadelphia: University of Pennsylvania Press, 1988), Ellen Chesler's *Woman of Valor: Margaret Sanger and the Birth Control Movement in America* (New York: Anchor Books, 1993), and Thomas Brown's *Dorothea Dix: New England Reformer* (Cambridge: Harvard University Press, 1998) all speak to the important place nursing held in these women's lives. Jane Robinson's *Mary Seacole: The Most Famous Black Woman of the Victorian Age* (New York: Carroll and Graf, 2004) brings the work of this Jamaican healer out from the glare of Nightingale's lamp. Naomi Rogers's *Healer from the Outback: Sister Elizabeth Kenny, Polio and American Medicine, 1940–1952* (New York: Oxford University Press, in press) considers the way appropriations of parts of nursing strengthened Kenny's challenge to medical orthodoxy. And, as Nella Larsen's literary reputation has undergone a late-twentieth-century renaissance, her life and work has been the subject of two biographies: Thadious Davis's *Nella Larsen, Novelist of the Harlem Renaissance: A Woman's Life Unveiled* (Baton Rouge: Louisiana State University Press, 1994) and George Hutchinson's *In Search of Nella Larsen: A Biography of the Color Line* (Cambridge: Belknap, 2006). My own interpretation borrows more heavily from Hutchinson, who sharply castigates those like Davis who would demean Larsen's decision to return to nursing when she emerged from seclusion. Instead, he sees it as a sign of strength.

We can finally look beyond Florence Nightingale if we seek fully developed stories of individual nurses and important work. Judith Godden's *Lucy Osburn, A Lady Displaced: Florence Nightingale's Envoy to Australia* (Sydney [AU] University Press, 2006) helps wean us as we make the transition. The best works in this genre use lives of nurses to complicate or challenge received wisdom about broader historical themes. Melanie Beals Goan's *Mary Breckinridge: The Frontier Nursing Service & Rural Health in Appalachia* (Chapel Hill: University of North Carolina Press, 2008) takes on those who would dismiss the work of Appalachian women reformers as, at best, ineffective and, at worst, destructive, and presents a portrait of achievement within a context of limitations. Similarly, Marjorie Feld's *Lillian Wald: A Biography* (Chapel Hill: University of North Carolina Press, 2009) takes issue with the conventional assumption about the American Progressive movement's Anglo-Protestant origins by locating Wald's work in the Jewish ethnic landscape of her time and place. But there are many more stories waiting to be told and ideas to be developed. Possible subjects might be found in anthologies carefully constructed by those keenly aware that nurses have not been well represented in ones about other notable American men and women. Those of note include Martin Kaufman's *Dictionary of American Nursing Biography* (Westport, CT: Greenwood, 1988) and Vern L. Bullough's three-volume *American Nursing: A Biographical Dictionary* (New York: Garland, 1988, 1992, 2000).

I join some few others in believing that specifically commissioned histories—most often of associations wishing to document their accomplishments or schools of nursing celebrating particular anniversaries—remain an important and underutilized source. Obviously, my own work acknowledges my debt to alumnae associations who painstakingly created the data I used in my analyses. There are as many of these books as there are states and associations, and I am forever indebted to Roberta West's *History of Nursing in Pennsylvania* (Harrisburg: Pennsylvania Nurses Association, 1926). These books, as a genre, deserve their own analysis for what they might suggest about nursing's sense of self and place. But the best of these individual histories stand as models for how one balances the tensions between data and critical analyses and how one engages audiences bringing different perspectives and expectations to the work. I have particularly enjoyed the way Barbara Brodie used pictures to tell a story in *Mr. Jefferson's Nurses: The University of Virginia School of Nursing, 1901–2001* (Charlottesville: University of Virginia Press, 2000), and how Marilyn Flood used documents in her *Promise on Parnassus: The First Century of the UCSF School of Nursing* (San Francisco: UCSF Nursing Press, 2007).

Lamps of the Prairie: A History of Nursing in Kansas (1942), commissioned by the Kansas State Nurses Association and compiled by the Writers' Program of the Depression-era Works Project Administration, still stands as one of the most important models of this kind of history. It might have languished in relative obscurity, however, had it not been rescued by a reprint series of seminal works in the history of American nursing edited by Susan Reverby and published by Garland through the 1980s. In this series, Barbara Melosh introduced readers to an array of evocative short stories about nurses in *American Nurses in Fiction: An Anthology of Short Stories* (1984). Darlene Clark Hine created a compelling collection of documents that have rarely been used in most accounts of nursing history in *Black Women in the Nursing Profession: A Documentary History* (1985). Reverby herself assembled the reports of an innovative and unusual nursing initiative in *The East Harlem Health Center Demonstration: An Anthology of Pamphlets* (1985). And Karen Buhler-Wilkerson's *Nursing and the Public's Health: An Anthology of Sources* (1989) brought together the seminal articles, surveys, and reports that defined the new field of public health nursing practice. We can look back in time to other anthologies, particularly Annie L. Austin's *A History of Nursing Sourcebook* (New York: Putnam, 1957), a large collection of sources that served as the basis for her own history of nursing. Unfortunately, we cannot yet look ahead to new ones—to ones that will reflect new areas of interest, newly discovered sources, new themes, and the too often invisible actors who have provided most of nursing's care.

For all the histories of schools of nursing, we still know relatively little about the complicated world of nursing education as it worked its way from training schools to universities and from granting diplomas to now conferring doctoral degrees. There are some notable exceptions. Theresa E. Christy's *Cornerstone for Nursing Education: A History of the Division of Nursing Education of Teachers College, Columbia University, 1899–1947* (1969) creates a vivid picture of an institution that played such a pivotal role in the history of nursing; and Patricia Haase's *The Origins and Rise of Associate Degree Nursing Education* (1990) tells of the transformation in nursing education that faculty at Teachers College helped create in post–World War II America—albeit unintendedly. But the history of education in nursing provides fertile ground for exploring issues in higher education in general. To my mind, it provides a perfect lens through which to consider the ways in which race and class intersected as private and public institutions decided which aspects of nursing education they would support and which they would ignore.

I could go on about what more we need to explore in the history of nursing. We need to know more about the experiences of minorities in nursing. We need to know more about practice and practice politics. But instead, I turn to the remarkable resources available to scholars interested in these and other issues in this particular, and admittedly small, field. The American Nursing History Archives at Boston University's Gotlieb Archival Research Center holds the official records of the American Nurses Association and the personal papers of many of the formal leaders associated with it. The Barbara Bates Center for the History of Nursing at the University of Pennsylvania, the Center for Nursing Historical Inquiry at the University of Virginia, and the Foundation of the New York State Nurses Association Center for Nursing History boast superb collections of records about more local nursing institutions and organizations. More importantly, they make a concerted effort to be more inclusive in their collecting policies. Their holdings do tell stories of nursing leaders. But they also tell stories of a much more diverse array of individuals with different kinds of contributions to their work and to their communities.

The most exciting sources, I think, have yet to be discovered. Nursing, as I have written, is rooted in and of its communities, and many of the sources I have used are embedded in other kinds of collections scattered throughout the country.

Modern technology made my historical research possible. Specialized search engines mining online data bases uncovered diaries, letters, and oral histories that would otherwise have passed unnoticed. I am not even sure that one still needs access to search engines like WORLDCAT. A simple search for "oral histories of black nurses," for example, yielded a rich array of sources collected by different kinds of groups wanting to document different kinds of experiences. I may never see an imagined future where a historian of nursing need not leave home or office to construct a story. However, I do see a future in which technology makes nurses and nursing more visible and encourages more people to bring their own questions about policy and practice to the fascinating world of the care of the sick in their particular communities of interest.

Page numbers in *italics* refer to figures and tables.

nursing leaders: attraction of candidates for training and, 89–90; in 1940s, 132; small schools and, 106–7; in South, 137–38, 223n. 7

Nutting, Adelaide, 36, 38, 70

Packard, John, 21
Parramore, Beatrice, 120
Partridge, Ruth, 101–2
paying for nursing, 7–9, 24
Pease, Nell Peckens, 41
Peck, (Louise) Arline, *91, 99*
Pennsylvania Hospital Training School for Nurses, 22–23
Philadelphia General Hospital, *Nursing Procedure Book,* 47
Philippines, nurses from, 171
Phillips, Harriet, 1, 66
physicians: knowledge of, 21, 52; protocols of, 42–43; thinking, 6, 10–12, 15–18; trained nurses and, 20–21; women as, 12–15, 26, 50, 58, 181
place of training and medical content, 39–41
polygamy/plural marriage, 83, 84, 90, 92
Powell, Alice, 98–99
power: at Grady, 111–12; knowledge and, 141; nursing leaders and, 50–51; Preston on, 14; sick nursing and, 5; of trained nurses, 16–17, 25–26
practice of medicine in twentieth century, 166–67
Prescott, Josephine Pitman, 136
Preston, Ann, 12, 13–15
private duty nurses, 56–60, 118, 164–65
private nursing, 61
professionalism: content and character as defining, 28–29, 30, 38–41; idea of, 134–38; integration in North Carolina and, 156; LPN category and, 149–50; NCSNA and, 140, 149–50; SANRN and, 145
protocols, 42–43
public health nursing: expansion of field of, 64–68; influential white women and, 123–24; life and work of, 68–72; racial discounting and, 66

public health system: in Atlanta, 109; in Georgia, 118–20
public perceptions of nursing, 122–23, 181–82
public space, hospitals as, 24–25
Putman, Charles, 15–16

race: Civil War nursing and, 9–10; discounting of in public health nursing, 66; in Georgia, 129–30; Glover and, 69–70; hiring nurses and, 7–8; of male nurses, 161–62, *187, 188, 189;* marital status of nurses and, *163, 164,* 174–76, *175, 190, 191, 192;* medical content of training and, 39; in nursing in early twentieth-century, 160–65, *187, 188;* nursing in South and, 107, 122–23, 124–27, 141–42; opportunities for advancement and, 74–75, 120; registration battles and, 116–17; SANRN and, 143–46; segregation and, 114–15; sick nursing and, 4, 26; training schools and, 111, 113
registered nursing: battles over, 115–17; pathways to, 170, 177–78
"responsible" nurses, Preston on, 13–15
Reverby, Susan, xvii–xviii, 9, 52
Riddle, Estelle Massey, 141–42, 157
Robb, Isabel Hampton, 33–35, 38, 42, 48–49
Rockefeller Foundation, 118, 123, 127, 132, 140
Roosevelt, Eleanor, 132
Rosenwald Foundation, 118, 131–32
Rosner, Lisa, 9

Salt Lake City, 85–86
Sandberg, Marilla (Fitzgerald), *91,* 101
San Francisco, *56, 66*
sanitary knowledge, 3, 6, 7, 19, 25
SANRN. *See* State Association of Negro Registered Nurses
Schissel, Carla, 116
school nurses, 65–66, 119
Schultz, Jane, 9
science content in training schools, 35–39